# HELICOBACTER PYLORI

# DEADLY DISEASES AND EPIDEMICS

Anthrax

Antibiotic-resistant Bacteria

Avian Flu

Botulism

Campylobacteriosis

Cervical Cancer

Cholera

Ebola

Encephalitis

*Escherichia coli* Infections

Gonorrhea

Hantavirus Pulmonary Syndrome

*Helicobacter pylori*

Hepatitis

Herpes

HIV/AIDS

Infectious Fungi

Influenza

Legionnaires' Disease

Leprosy

Lyme Disease

Lung Cancer

Mad Cow Disease (Bovine Spongiform Encephalopathy)

Malaria

Meningitis

Mononucleosis

Pelvic Inflammatory Disease

Plague

Polio

Prostate Cancer

Rabies

*Salmonella*

SARS

Smallpox

*Streptococcus* (Group A)

*Staphylococcus aureus* Infections

Syphilis

Toxic Shock Syndrome

Tuberculosis

Tularemia

Typhoid Fever

West Nile Virus

# HELICOBACTER PYLORI

## Shawna L. Fleming, Ph.D.

FOUNDING EDITOR
The Late **I. Edward Alcamo**
Distinguished Teaching Professor of Microbiology,
SUNY Farmingdale

FOREWORD BY
**David Heymann**
World Health Organization

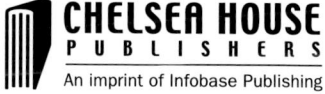

**CHELSEA HOUSE**
P U B L I S H E R S
An imprint of Infobase Publishing

**Helicobacter pylori**

Chelsea House
An imprint of Infobase Publishing
132 West 31st Street
New York NY 10001

**Library of Congress Cataloging-in-Publication Data**

Fleming, Shawna L.
  Helicobacter pylori / Shawna L. Fleming ; foreword by David Heyman.
      p. cm.—(Deadly diseases and epidemics)
  Includes bibliographical references and index.
  ISBN 0-7910-8681-X (hc : alk. paper)
  1. Helicobacter pylori infections—Juvenile literature. 2. Helicobacter pylori—Juvenile literature. I. Title. II. Series.
  RC 840.H38F54 2006
  616.3'3014—dc22                                                                     2006015153

Chelsea House books are available at special discounts when purchased in bulk quantities for businesses, associations, institutions, or sales promotions. Please call our Special Sales Department in New York at (212) 967-8800 or (800) 322-8755.

You can find Chelsea House on the World Wide Web at http://www.chelseahouse.com

Series design by Terry Mallon
Cover design by Takeshi Takahashi

Printed in the United States of America

Bang EJB 10 9 8 7 6 5 4 3 2 1

This book is printed on acid-free paper.

All links and Web addresses were checked and verified to be correct at the time of publication. Because of the dynamic nature of the Web, some addresses and links may have changed since publication and may no longer be valid.

# Table of Contents

# Foreword

**In the 1960s, many of the infectious diseases that had terrorized** generations were tamed. After a century of advances, the leading killers of Americans both young and old were being prevented with new vaccines or cured with new medicines. The risk of death from pneumonia, tuberculosis (TB), meningitis, influenza, whooping cough, and diphtheria declined dramatically. New vaccines lifted the fear that summer would bring polio, and a global campaign was on the verge of eradicating smallpox worldwide. New pesticides like DDT cleared mosquitoes from homes and fields, thus reducing the incidence of malaria, which was present in the southern United States and which remains a leading killer of children worldwide. New technologies produced safe drinking water and removed the risk of cholera and other water-borne diseases. Science seemed unstoppable. Disease seemed destined to all but disappear.

But the euphoria of the 1960s has evaporated.

The microbes fought back. Those causing diseases like TB and malaria evolved resistance to cheap and effective drugs. The mosquito developed the ability to defuse pesticides. New diseases emerged, including AIDS, Legionnaire's, and Lyme disease. And diseases which had not been seen in decades re-emerged, as the hantavirus did in the Navajo Nation in 1993. Technology itself actually created new health risks. The global transportation network, for example, meant that diseases like West Nile virus could spread beyond isolated regions and quickly become global threats. Even modern public health protections sometimes failed, as they did in 1993 in Milwaukee, Wisconsin, resulting in 400,000 cases of the digestive system illness cryptosporidiosis. And, more recently, the threat from smallpox, a disease believed to be completely eradicated, has returned along with other potential bioterrorism weapons such as anthrax.

The lesson is that the fight against infectious diseases will never end.

In our constant struggle against disease, we as individuals have a weapon that does not require vaccines or drugs, and that is the warehouse of knowledge. We learn from the history of science that "modern" beliefs can be wrong. In this series of books, for example, you will learn that diseases like syphilis were once thought to be caused by eating potatoes. The invention of the microscope set science on the right path. There are more positive lessons from history. For example, smallpox was eliminated by vaccinating everyone who had come in contact with an infected person. This "ring" approach to smallpox control is still the preferred method for confronting an outbreak, should the disease be intentionally reintroduced.

At the same time, we are constantly adding new drugs, new vaccines, and new information to the warehouse. Recently, the entire human genome was decoded. So too was the genome of the parasite that causes malaria. Perhaps by looking at the microbe and the victim through the lens of genetics we will be able to discover new ways to fight malaria, which remains the leading killer of children in many countries.

Because of advances in our understanding of such diseases as AIDS, entire new classes of antiretroviral drugs have been developed. But resistance to all these drugs has already been detected, so we know that AIDS drug development must continue.

Education, experimentation, and the discoveries that grow out of them are the best tools to protect health. Opening this book may put you on the path of discovery. I hope so, because new vaccines, new antibiotics, new technologies, and, most importantly, new scientists are needed now more than ever if we are to remain on the winning side of this struggle against microbes.

David Heymann
Executive Director
Communicable Diseases Section
World Health Organization
Geneva, Switzerland

# 1

# The Discovery
# of *Helicobacter pylori*

In his dream, Erik was battling a pack of animals that were gnawing through his stomach. However, when he awoke, he discovered that the burning, gnawing pain in his stomach wasn't a dream. The pain was familiar, and being awakened by it was nothing new. Erik leaned over and grabbed the bottle of Pepto Bismol on his night stand—his beverage of choice with most meals lately, and sometimes between meals. He had been under a ton of pressure, with the SATs looming and his parents worrying incessantly over his grades. Erik would be the first member of his Polish-immigrant family to go to college, and the pressure was on in a big way; he was stressing under all of the bragging and high expectations of his family.

He had also been feeling very tired lately, which he attributed to the fact that, along with studying hard for exams and classes, baseball season was starting. Between practice and the homework he hadn't had a lot of time for sleep, and hadn't exactly been eating well when he and his friends went for burgers and pizza after practice. His stomach had always annoyed him somewhat, but recently the pain had been getting worse, particularly after extremely spicy or acidic foods, which he loved. He had known when eating the chili dog and atomic salsa that evening that he would pay for it, but this was even worse than usual. He managed a few more hours of fitful sleep before he had to get ready for school, but when he tried to get up he felt dizzy and weak, and decided that he should see the doctor.

After undergoing a series of tests, it was determined that Erik had a bleeding ulcer, which the doctor told him was a condition that can occur

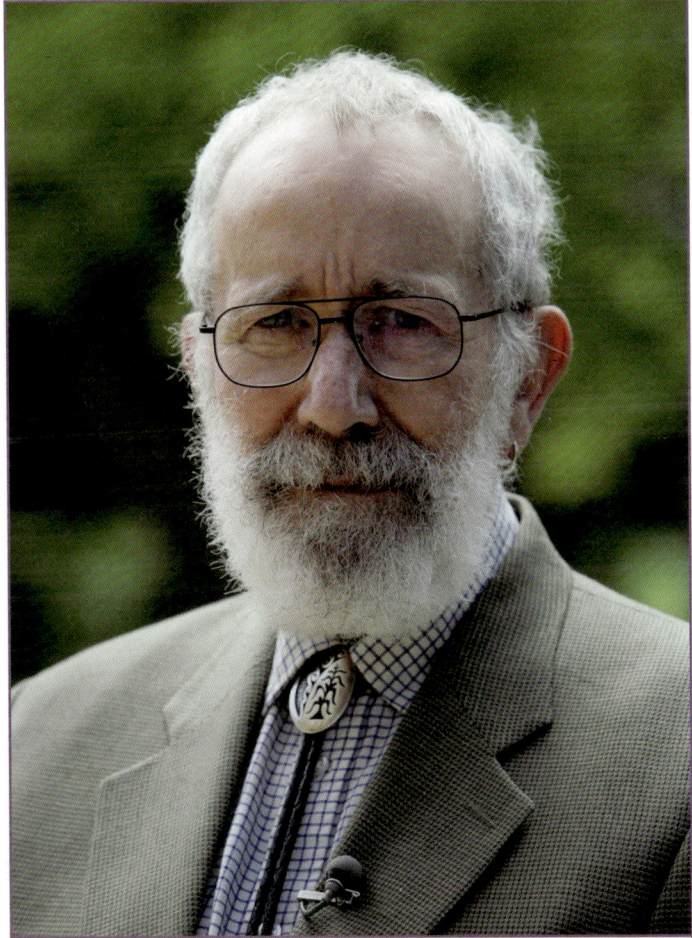

**Figure 1.1** Dr. Robbin Warren, winner of the 2005 Nobel Prize in Medicine. (©Ross Swansborough/epa/Corbis)

when an ulcer forms in the vicinity of a blood vessel, causing bleeding into the stomach. His father and grandfather had both had ulcers, so Erik wasn't surprised by the news. The x-ray showed that he had a spot about the size of a nickel in his stomach, while his blood tests revealed that he was both anemic and carried antibodies to the bacterium *Helicobacter pylori*, which

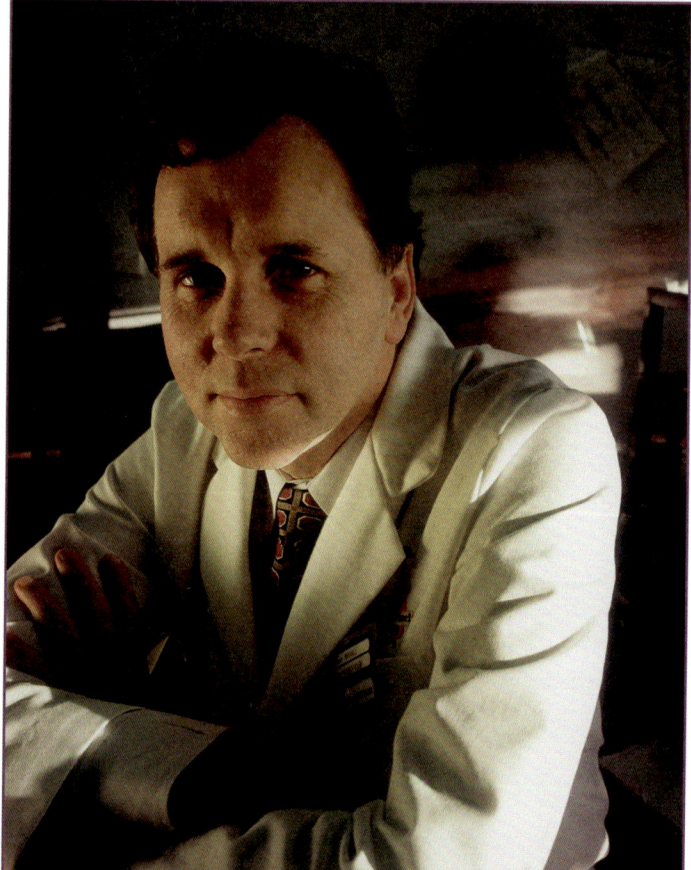

**Figure 1.2** Dr. Barry Marshall, winner of the 2005 Nobel Prize in Medicine. (©Tony McDonough/epa/Corbis)

is known to cause stomach ulcers. To Erik, the best news was that, given sufficient time and a full course of treatment, the condition was curable.

In October of 2005 the Nobel Prize in medicine was awarded to two Australian physicians, Dr. Robbin Warren and Dr. Barry Marshall (Figures 1.1 and 1.2), for the discovery of *Helicobacter pylori*, the organism that causes ulcers and other diseases of the upper digestive system. This was an extremely important discovery. *H. pylori* infection is one of the most common infectious diseases on earth, and is responsible for a tremendous amount of illness and suffering worldwide. Over half of the world's population is infected with this organism. In the United States alone (where the rate of infection is relatively low) there are over 6,500 ulcer-related deaths per year and over $6 billion lost in worker productivity as a result of ulcer-related illness. *H. pylori* is also believed to be the most important cause of stomach cancers, and the second-leading cause of cancer-related deaths worldwide. Over 90 percent of people who develop certain types of stomach cancer are infected with *H. pylori*.

As you will see from the story that follows, establishing the link between *H. pylori* and stomach ulcers was no easy task. The association between *H. pylori* and ulcer formation was one of the most controversial hypotheses in recent medical history, and as a result Warren and Marshall had many obstacles to overcome before *H. pylori* was accepted by the scientific and medical communities as a disease-causing organism. However, the tale of its discovery is a fascinating example of how good scientific detective work, and determination to forge ahead in the face of repeated rejections, can change the way that diseases are understood and treated.

## WHAT IS *HELICOBACTER PYLORI*?

*Helicobacter pylori* is a helical, or spiral-shaped, bacterium (Figure 1.3) that lives in the stomach. No one knows how long it has been working its mischief, but the best guess is that it has been around for several millennia. Infection with *H. pylori* is associated with a number of diseases including stomach and duodenal ulcers, as well as certain cancers. However, only a small fraction of infected people experience noticeable symptoms, and for that reason diagnosis of the infection is quite low when compared to the number of people who are actually

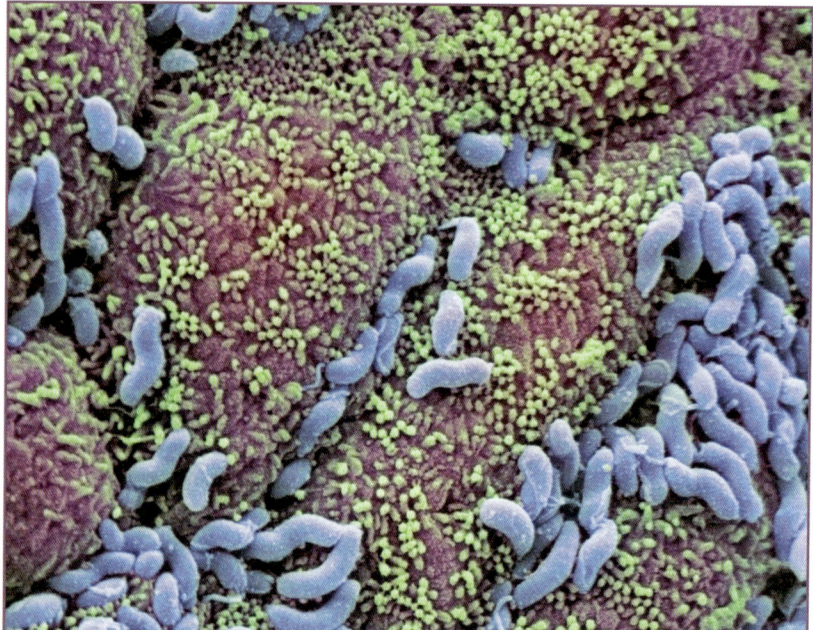

**Figure 1.3** This is a scanning electron micrograph image of *Helicobacter pylori* bacteria (in blue). These Gram-negative, rod-shaped bacteria are commonly found in the mucosal lining of the stomach of people with ulcers. (©David McCarthy/Photo Researchers, Inc.)

infected. Even in those who eventually develop ulcers, these symptoms—which include burping, nausea, and burning or aching in the stomach—are usually subtle and can be confused with other diseases. As a result, the infection often goes unde-tected for many years. It is precisely because *H. pylori* infection is not associated with a hallmark set of outward symptoms that it took centuries to establish the relationship between *H. pylori* infection and ulcers.

### *H. PYLORI*: PATHOGEN OR INNOCENT BYSTANDER?

What if you were told that headaches are caused by a germ that infected you as a baby, and that all you have to do to prevent yourself from ever getting another headache is to take antibiotics for a few weeks? Would you believe it? Probably not. What are some of the problems with that statement? You're probably thinking, "Everyone gets headaches," which is (mostly) true. You might also think, "How do you know that a germ causes headaches? What germ causes them?" and "Why didn't I get headaches when I was a baby?" Those are also good questions. But, in addition to being unconvinced by the argument, you might also have your own ideas based on your experience and what has become common social (if not exactly medical) knowledge. You might also think, "I know what causes my headaches! Stress!"

This is precisely what the many people who proposed the relationship between *H. pylori* infection and stomach ulcers came up against for decades—indeed, centuries—and it wasn't just the public who had to be convinced, it was the entire scientific community, the members of which have a great deal of experience studying and/or treating human disease. When a specific organism exists in many people, but only a few have symptoms of disease, it is difficult to prove that the organism, and not something else entirely, is causing the condition. Proving the association between an organism and a disease is particularly difficult when the symptoms are common to a number of different conditions. Stomach pain, nausea, and burning can be attributed to a variety of conditions such as food intolerance, acid reflux disease, or stomach viruses. Another problem is that the stomach is not an organ that a doctor can easily look at in order to make a diagnosis (internal examinations of the stomach are not often done unless a person's symptoms are severe). So, unlike a case of poison ivy on a person's skin (which can be seen), or a case in which it's possible to conduct a direct examination of a diseased organ, the physician has to rely on less direct measures to make a diagnosis. As a result, *H. pylori* infection has often been misdiagnosed in sick patients.

Under these circumstances the only way to convincingly prove that an organism is responsible for a particular disease, as opposed to being just an innocent bystander, is to reproduce the disease in a healthy person or an animal model. This, however, is very difficult to do in humans (doctors don't often intentionally make their patients sick), and, until recently, very little was known about animals that might be susceptible to *H.*

## A BRIEF INTRODUCTION TO BACTERIA

Bacteria are microscopic, single-celled organisms. Most bacteria are approximately a few microns (millionths of a meter [1 yard = 0.914 meters]) in length, and occupy a very wide range of habitats. Bacteria can be found inhabiting territories ranging from deep-sea vents to the tops of mountains to the frozen depths of glaciers. While bacteria have caused some of our most terrible diseases, most are completely harmless, and some are truly beneficial. For example, yogurt and cheese would certainly not be the same without bacteria, and some bacteria that inhabit the human intestinal tract manufacture products (such as vitamin K) that are essential for normal physiology.

Bacteria are also essential components of the ecosystem. By degrading dead material they recycle nutrients and minerals back into the environment. Some are even capable of taking nitrogen from the air, thereby replenishing soil with nitrogen that can be taken up by plants. However, certain bacteria such as *Yersinia pestis* (which causes the plague), *Clostridium botulinum* (which causes botulism), and *Vibrio cholerae* (which causes cholera) are also pathogenic and have been a source of suffering and death throughout human history. As opposed to viral infections, however, most bacterial infections can be treated with antibiotics, which has virtually eliminated many of mankind's most feared and fatal diseases from our everyday lives.

*pylori* infection and so could be used as experimental models. As you will see from the discussion that follows, establishing the relationship between H. *pylori* and stomach disease was very difficult; it took considerable ingenuity and persistence on the part of numerous scientists.

## A BRIEF HISTORY OF PEPTIC ULCER DISEASE AND THE DISCOVERY OF *H. PYLORI*

As with most diseases, recognition of the symptoms of ulcers (intense, gnawing stomach pain) preceded understanding of their causes. One of the first people to describe what a stomach ulcer looks like was the Italian physician Marcellus Donatus of Mantua in 1586, who identified one during an autopsy. Other descriptions of what appeared to be open, raw sores in the lining of the stomach (ulcers) soon followed; however, none of these observations shed much light on the causes of the disease itself. In fact, as late as the 1980s, physicians attributed the development of ulcers to a combination of diet and emotional factors, such as nervousness and stress. While these factors may indeed aggravate ulcers, one of the primary risk factors for developing an ulcer is now known to be H. *pylori* infection.

The first person thought to have described a *Helicobacter*-like bacterium living in the stomach of any animal was another Italian physician named Giulio Bizzozero, who presented his finding at a meeting of the Turin Medical Academy in 1892. In this presentation he described what he called "spirilli," or spiral organisms, which he observed in tissues taken from the stomachs of dogs. He described an organism of approximately 3-8 microns (or millionths of a meter ($\mu$M) [1 yard = 0.914 meters]) that contained between 3 and 7 coils and was found in the lumen, or cavity, of the mucus-secreting glands in the stomach. Considering that the microscopes available at that time were much less powerful than today's equipment, and that the techniques to preserve and stain tissues were not yet well developed, the fact that he managed to both observe these organisms in microscopically complex animal tissues, and accurately describe their physical structure and how they were distributed in the tissue, is rather amazing.

Nevertheless, Bizzozero's observation was viewed as only a mildly curious finding and, lacking any human data, the observation was essentially overlooked until recently. However, around the same time, a number of other scientists began to report seeing spiral organisms in the stomachs of humans. These bacteria were described from autopsy and surgical specimens of patients with ulcers and gastric cancer. While of interest to many scientists and doctors, it could not be demonstrated that the bacteria were responsible for causing the disease.

This prompted a physician named Dr. Eddy D. Palmer, during his tenure at Walter Reed Army Hospital, to devise a method of removing the bacteria from the stomach using a vacuum tube apparatus, which he felt would allow him to isolate the bacteria from intact tissue without contamination from other sources. After examining over 1,000 patients, however, he was unable to recover any bacteria. He reported his observations in 1954 and concluded that, in living organisms, the stomach cannot be colonized by bacteria. Given the fact that the stomach is essentially a bag of acid, he believed that the environment of the human stomach is not capable of supporting bacterial growth, and that previous reports of bacterial infection of human stomach tissue were the result of contamination introduced during removal of the tissue.

The general consensus at this time was that ulcers resulted from an imbalance between the protective functions of the stomach (mucus secretion) and the secretion of acid and digestive enzymes. The theory was that if the amount of protective mucus wasn't enough to overcome the activity of the acid produced by the stomach, ulcers would be formed. It was also thought that excessive nervousness or stress caused an increase in the acid production of the stomach, which led to a breakdown of the normal tissue (the so-called "acid hypothesis" of ulcer production, which drugs like Tagamet were developed to treat).

This idea was very appealing, since it was mostly confirmed by the appearance of tissue taken from people who suffered from ulcers. The tissue did look as though it was being digested by its own secretions, and for anyone who has ever gotten pickle juice in a paper cut, it also explained the intense burning pain that ulcer sufferers experienced. And there did seem to be a relationship between stress and severity of disease; yet it wasn't clear whether the stress caused the disease or the disease caused the stress.

Within the medical establishment, the idea that the stomach was an impossibly hostile environment for bacteria persisted for over 35 years. However, in 1954, at about the time that Dr. Palmer published his report on the sterility of the stomach, reports were also beginning to surface that several doctors had successfully cured their patients' ulcers with antibiotic therapy. Because antibiotics are drugs that work by interfering with processes or molecules that are specifically used by bacteria, it was concluded by these physicians that bacteria were the cause of many ulcers. Antibiotics were a fairly new type of medicine at this time, though, and most people didn't know how to interpret the results. Also, since many of the reports were anecdotal, meaning that they were not the result of carefully controlled experiments, most scientists and physicians disregarded the observations as inconclusive.

One of the chief advocates for the use of antibiotic therapy for the treatment of ulcers was a Greek physician named John Lykoudis, who in 1958 cured his own ulcers by undergoing a round of antibiotic treatment. He then tried this therapy on some of his patients, many of whom were also cured by the treatment. In an effort to improve his therapy, he experimented with a number of different drug combinations and finally arrived at a formula that he claimed cured 100 percent of the patients he treated. Encouraged by his results in human subjects, he sought governmental approval for his treatment regimen, but was repeatedly denied, even after submitting the names and addresses of over 12,000 patients whom he claimed to have cured! Over the next few decades similar stories emerged from Russia, England, and China, but as before no one was able to overcome the prevailing notion in the medical community that it was acid, not bacteria, that caused ulcers.

It wasn't until the mid-1980s that Warren and Marshall finally succeeded in convincing the medical community about the relationship between *H. pylori* and the formation of ulcers. As you will see, this was no simple task. It took much determination, hard work, and some rather unorthodox methods to accomplish this feat.

Dr. Warren, a pathologist in Western Australia, first noticed *Helicobacter* organisms on his birthday in June of 1979. By this time technical advances in medicine had changed the way that diseases were diagnosed. The widespread availability of the fiberoptic endoscope, an instrument inserted into the stomach via the mouth, allowed physicians to collect high-quality tissue specimens that they could examine microscopically (Figure 1.4). This greatly increased the ability of pathologists to view the fine details of tissue specimens.

While examining a biopsy specimen of tissue taken from a person with chronic gastritis (inflammation of the stomach lining), Dr. Warren noticed fine, blue lines on the surface of the mucosa, the cells lining the stomach, in areas that were clearly damaged and inflamed. At higher magnification, he observed what appeared to be numerous small bacteria, which he described in the patient's pathology report. Intrigued by this observation, which flew in the face of all of his previous medical training about the growth of bacteria in the stomach, he continued to search for bacteria in other specimens that he received. After viewing a large number of these inflamed, bacteria-containing tissues, he became

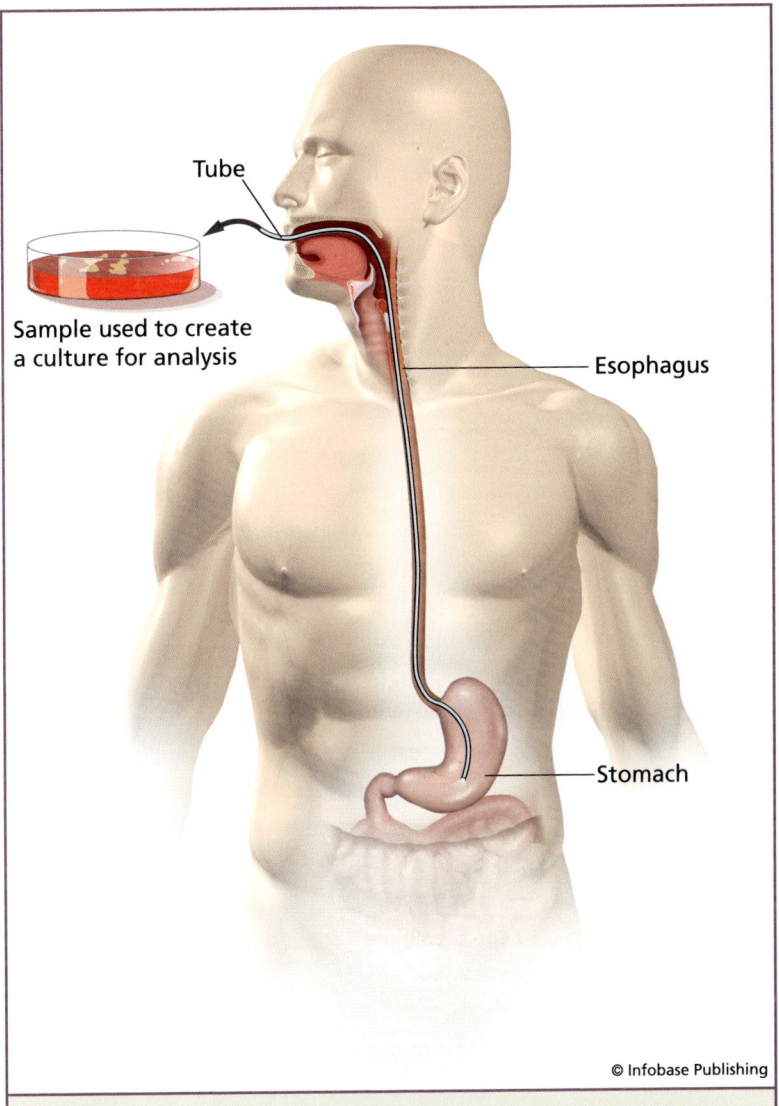

Tube

Sample used to create
a culture for analysis

Esophagus

Stomach

© Infobase Publishing

**Figure 1.4** Diagram of an endoscope, an instrument used to
view the inside of the stomach. An endoscope is inserted down
the throat into the stomach. A camera and a biopsy instrument
enable surgeons to view and remove diseased tissue for examination by a pathologist, who renders a diagnosis.

convinced that the infections were the cause of the inflammation and damage that he saw in the mucosa. This discovery was
quite puzzling! He couldn't understand why he hadn't heard of
this before, so he went to the library to do some research. After
considerable searching, he happened across a published
description of similar specimens taken from human tissue and
began to work in earnest to understand the role of these bacteria in diseases of the stomach.

## HELICOBACTERS IN ANTIQUITY

Chile's Atacama Desert is one of the driest places on earth.
In many parts of this region, rainfall has never been recorded.
Yet, despite its harsh climate, it is also one of the most spec-
tacularly beautiful landscapes imaginable. Otherworldly rock
formations and expansive salt lakes are interspersed with
regions in which bright blue skies and rugged, rocky peaks
frame a terrain of billowy, bright sand that is almost completely unmarred by animal or plant life.

While perhaps not a great place to plan a family vacation,
the Atacama Desert is an excellent place to search for mummies! It has in fact proven a veritable treasure-trove of mummified human remains, some of which are many thousands of
years old. In this highly arid climate, corpses tend to dehy-
drate rather than decay, providing some of the most intact
specimens available. Unlike Egyptian mummies, which underwent elaborate mummification procedures prior to being
placed in their tombs, these specimens have mummified without extensive handling, and for that reason their internal
organs are often largely intact. The scarcity of human and animal life has allowed these specimens to rest relatively undis-
turbed for centuries.

Dr. Marvin Allison and his colleague at Virginia Common-
wealth University in Richmond, Virginia, Dr. Enrique Gerszten,

## H. PYLORI: NOT JUST AN INNOCENT BYSTANDER

In 1981 Barry Marshall came to work with Dr. Warren. They began a clinical study of patients who were referred for endoscopy. Using samples of tissue taken during the endoscopy procedure, they attempted to grow the infection-causing organism in the laboratory. Thinking the bacterium to be a type of *Campylobacter*, they attempted to grow their specimens under conditions appropriate for that organism, but failed

have spent their careers studying the undoing of our ancient ancestors. They have been particularly interested in understanding the diseases from which ancient people suffered, and how these diseases have spread through human civilizations over time. These scientists employ a sophisticated combination of archaeological and modern molecular methods to discover how these people lived and died.

So what diseases did our ancient ancestors contract? According to Drs. Allison and Gerszten, they suffered from many of the same conditions that we currently battle! Using their expertise in performing anatomical examinations, similar to those used during modern-day autopsies, they found such commonplace conditions as emphysema, breast cancer, and pneumonia.

By applying cutting-edge molecular biology methods, they also identified several infectious diseases within these ancient specimens. Using bits of feces from the intestines of 1,700-year-old mummies, they discovered that our ancient relatives not only suffered from the same modern-day diarrheal parasites, such as *Cryptosporidium* and *Giardia*, but they were also infected with *Helicobacter pylori*, providing the first evidence that humans and *Helicobacters* have had a very, very long history together!

repeatedly. Eventually, another scientist recommended they try a recently-developed technique known as microaerophilic culture, which uses a chamber with low oxygen content, similar to what the bacteria would encounter in the stomach.

After many months of trying to isolate the bacterium from fresh biopsy specimens, it was only accidentally that they were finally able to obtain a culture of *H. pylori*. The team had been waiting just one to two days before discarding specimens. But, over the Easter holiday in 1982 someone on Marshall and Warren's team inadvertently left a culture plate in the incubator for five days. Upon returning the following Tuesday, they found a group of small, transparent colonies growing in the culture dish, making this the first successful attempt to culture the organism in the laboratory!

Finding and isolating the germ was only the first step in demonstrating that it was actually responsible for causing human disease, and not simply an innocent bystander. Marshall and Warren studied over 65 patients with the bacteria, and almost all had microscopic evidence of inflammation in their stomachs. The frequency of infection among those with ulcers was nearly 90 percent! While this piece of information was highly suggestive, it still did not prove that the bacterium actually caused disease, since Marshall and Warren couldn't really know how many people in the population had the bacterium but didn't have the disease.

Marshall and Warren then began a series of experiments in which they attempted to infect young pigs with the bacterium; the goal was to determine whether the disease could be re-created in the animals. If so, it would demonstrate that the bacterium actually causes disease. Pigs have been known to suffer from ulcers and are large enough to undergo endoscopy, so the two researchers inoculated the animals with the bacteria and waited. After many rounds of endoscopy, no inflammation in the pigs' stomachs was observed, nor were the scientists able to re-isolate the organism. After a time, the pigs outgrew the endoscopes, which, having been built for humans, were too short to reach the stomach of a full-grown pig. That, combined with the fact that the pigs became too difficult to catch and anesthetize, forced Marshall and Warren to abandon their experiments.

At this point they were running out of options. So in a last-ditch effort, Dr. Marshall decided to test his hypothesis on himself. He underwent an endoscopy to collect a biopsy specimen of his uninfected tissue, and then swallowed a sample of a live bacterial culture that he had isolated from one of his patients. After seven days he began to notice symptoms and, after a few days of vomiting, underwent another endoscopic exam. The tissue retrieved from Dr. Marshall's stomach had many of the hallmark features present in his patients' samples: inflammatory cells and loads of bacteria! The results of this experiment demonstrated for the first time that the bacterium was not simply an innocent bystander—it was capable of causing gastritis, which was, Marshall and Warren believed, the first step on the road to ulcer formation.

It is now well established that *H. pylori* is a pathogen and is associated not only with ulcers, but also with stomach cancer and gastric lymphoma (another type of cancer). The evidence is so strong, in fact, that in 1994 *H. pylori* was declared a Class 1 (or definite) carcinogen by the International Agency for Research on Cancer (IARC), a subset of the World Health Organization.

# 2

# The Anatomy and Physiology of Digestion: What Happens to the Food that You Eat?

Virtually all living organisms, apart from plants and certain **photosynthetic** bacteria and algae, must acquire their energy from outside of their bodies. Some single-celled organisms that live in a highly nutritive environment, like the intestinal tract of an animal, may obtain nutrition simply by absorbing it from that environment; however, for most multicellular organisms, the body wall is too thick to permit efficient diffusion of nutrients to the cells of the organism's interior. These organisms must therefore obtain nutrition by eating. The digestive system is the group of organs that processes food into nutrients that can be used by the body.

Animals require nutrients for growth, repair, and to supply energy for basic functions like breathing and maintaining body temperature. In order to reach the innermost parts of the body, nutrients must leave the digestive system and enter the blood stream. To do this, the food must be broken into individual molecules small enough to pass through the intestinal tract, where they are taken up by small blood vessels called **capillaries**. The chief function of the digestive system is therefore to transfer ingested nutrients from the outside to the inside of the body. A second major function is to eliminate undigested matter and other wastes. To accomplish these tasks, a number of physical and chemical processes must be performed to break the food into its component parts, absorb and transport the nutrients, and expel what remains.

## THE ANATOMY OF DIGESTION

The digestive system can be thought of as a disassembly line on which food is broken into pieces small enough to squeeze through the spaces between the cells of the intestine. During this process, food is moved along a conveyor belt (your digestive system) from station to station (or, in this case, organ to organ), being taken apart as it passes through.

The organs of the digestive system (Figure 2.1) are essentially cylindrical structures that join together to form one continuous tube that extends from the mouth to the anus. These are the machines in the disassembly line that mechanically and chemically break down food and eliminate waste. The organs involved include the mouth, **pharynx** (throat), **esophagus**, **stomach** (Figure 2.2), **duodenum**, small intestine, large intestine (consisting of the **ascending colon**, **transverse colon**, and **descending colon**) and the **rectum**. This sequence of organs is sometimes called the alimentary canal. In addition to this 'heavy equipment' in the disassembly factory, there are also numerous smaller accessory structures and organs that aid in the disassembly process, including the teeth, **salivary glands**, **liver** and **gall bladder**, and **pancreas**.

The disassembly machine kicks into high gear when food is taken into the mouth. The teeth, tongue, and salivary glands provide the first stage of the mechanical disassembly by grinding and mashing the food into a semi-liquid paste. Once food is thoroughly **masticated** (chewed) and mixed with saliva, it can be swallowed. Swallowing, or **deglutition**, involves the coordinated actions of several organs that act in synchrony to move the **bolus**, or mouthful of food, into the esophagus. During swallowing, the tongue compresses food against the roof of the mouth, pushing the food backward into the pharynx. How-

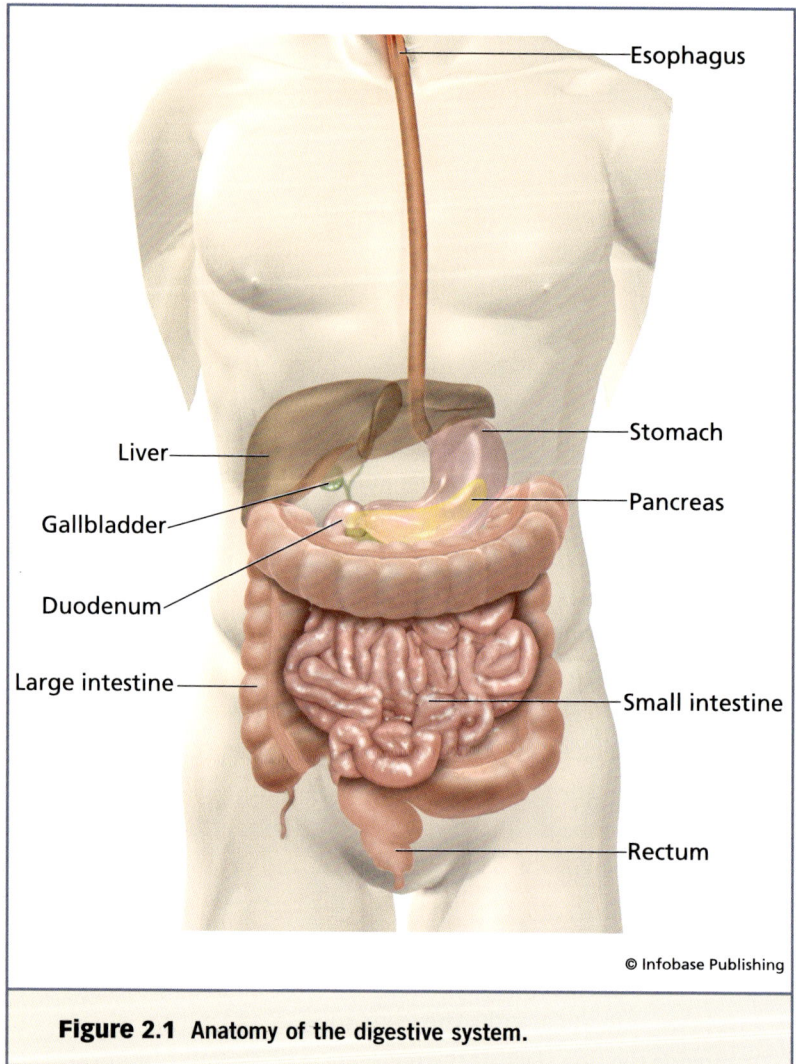

**Figure 2.1 Anatomy of the digestive system.**

ever, for food to enter the esophagus (the conveyor belt that transports food to the stomach), it must bypass the **trachea**, or windpipe. This is accomplished through a structure called the **epiglottis**, a trap door over the entrance to the airway that snaps shut each time something is swallowed, thus preventing materials from entering the respiratory system.

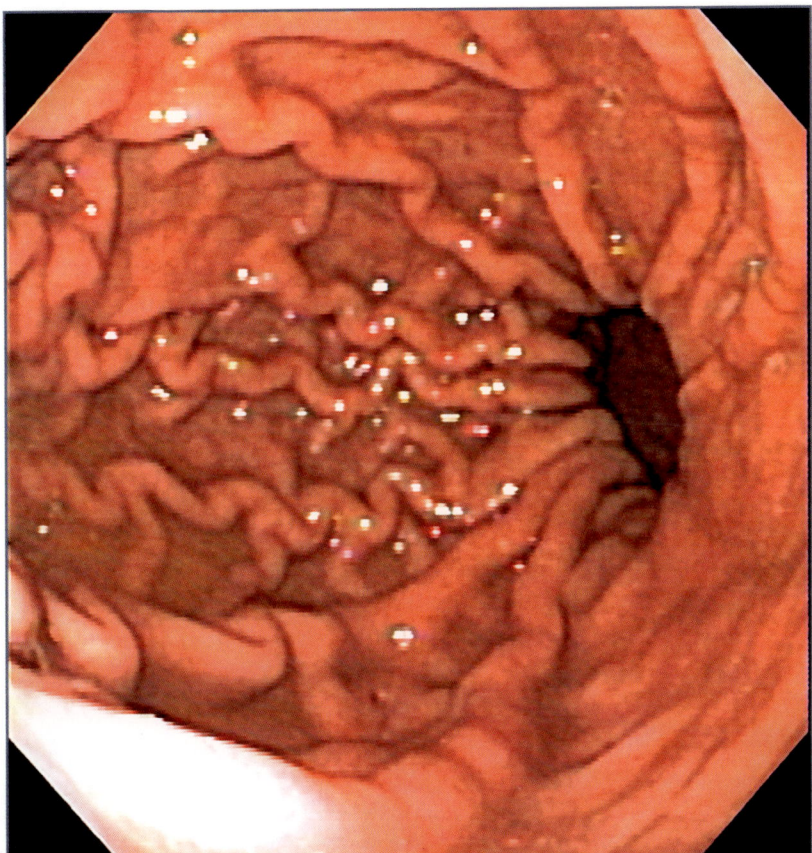

**Figure 2.2** The body of the stomach (as seen through an endo-scope) contains rugal folds, which secrete mucus, acid, and enzymes necessary for digestion. (©David Musher/Photo Researchers, Inc.)

Once food enters the esophagus, it is conveyed toward the stomach by a series of muscular contractions called **peristaltic waves**. These motions, generated by the contraction of numerous muscular fibers that encircle and line the walls of the esophagus, transport the food down to the opening of the stomach. When food reaches the stomach it must pass through an opening called the **gastroesophageal sphincter**, a muscular

(*continued on page 30*)

# DIGESTION OF PROTEINS

Proteins are large molecules made up of strings of amino acids, which, for the most part, are composed of carbon (C), hydrogen (H), oxygen (O), and nitrogen (N). Amino acids are connected to one another by a chemical structure known as a peptide bond (Figure 2.3, Figure 2.4), in which the nitrogen on the left side of one amino acid joins to the carbon on the right side of the next amino acid. This creates a linear string of amino acids that then folds back on itself, forming very specific structures. A protein's structure is important in determining its function. Proteins perform an enormous array of functions inside cells; virtually every type of protein performs a specific and different role in the organism. Proteins compose the cell's skeleton and aid in molecular communication (within and between cells, and from one

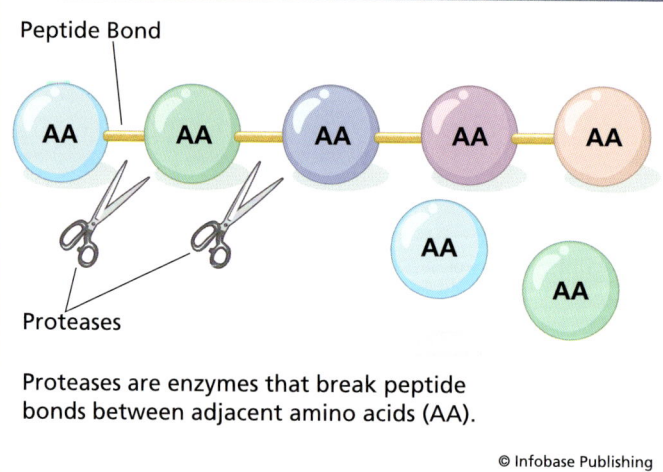

Peptide Bond

Proteases

Proteases are enzymes that break peptide bonds between adjacent amino acids (AA).

© Infobase Publishing

**Figure 2.3** Proteases are enzymes that break peptide bonds between adjacent amino acids.

organ to another). Enzymes are also proteins; they promote chemical reactions inside and outside of cells.

One class of digestive enzyme, called a protease, digests proteins by cutting the peptide bond between adjacent amino acids. This frees amino acids from one another and allows them to be absorbed by the intestinal tract and re-used by the body.

The liver can make most amino acids; however, the body cannot manufacture all amino acids, so it is necessary for people to acquire some of them from their diet. These are called essential amino acids. Proteases in the intestinal tract re-supply the body with essential amino acids, to replenish the supply depleted by the body's various metabolic processes.

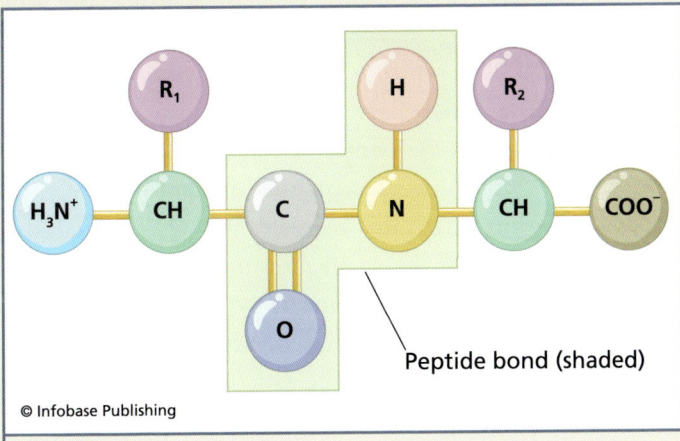

Peptide bond (shaded)

© Infobase Publishing

**Figure 2.4** The chemical structure of amino acids joined in a peptide bond. $R_1$ and $R_2$ are generic designations for other chemical structures. Amino acids are distinguished from one another by the chemical structure of their "R" groups.

(*continued from page 27*)
constriction that opens to permit passage of food into the stomach and then closes to prevent the backflow of stomach content into the esophagus.

The stomach is a large, washing machine-like organ located in the upper left side of the abdominal cavity, just beneath the diaphragm. In the sequence of organs that constitute the digestive tract, the stomach lies between the esophagus and small intestine. The stomach is joined to the esophagus at a region called the cardia, which is situated just beyond the gastroesophageal sphincter. The stomach can be thought of as having two sections: the **body** and the **antrum** (Figure 2.5). The fundus, a region located at the top of the stomach's body, is often discussed separately in scientific textbooks, but physiologically functions as part of the body. The stomach's body is the region in which mucus, acid, and digestive enzymes are produced. When food enters the stomach, it triggers powerful muscular contractions that "agitate" or churn the food like a washing machine, causing further breakdown of the food into smaller and smaller pieces. After the stomach, the next station is the intestinal tract, which is the transport and distribution center of the disassembly line.

The lower part of the stomach is joined to the small intestine via the duodenum, a structure of approximately 10 inches (25 cm) in length that regulates the rate at which the stomach empties into the small intestine. Partially digested food, called **chyme**, flowing from the stomach to the duodenum must pass through another muscular gate called the **pyloric sphincter**, or **pylorus**. The rate of flow into the duodenum is controlled by hormonal and nervous signals, and by the volume and chemical composition of the chyme, as will be described below.

The duodenum is attached to the small intestine, a tube of about 20 feet (approximately 6.1 meters) in length, which contains two parts: the **jejunum**, the upper segment of the small intestine, and the **ileum**, the lower segment. The duodenum is

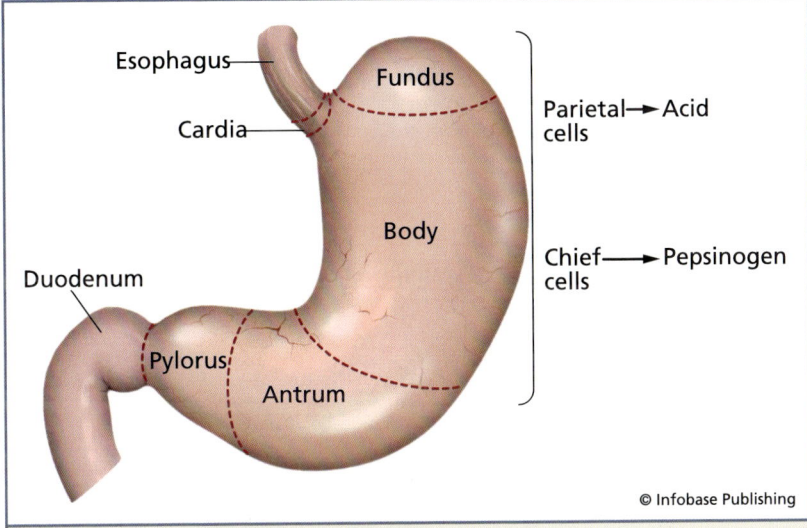

**Esophagus**

**Fundus**

**Cardia**

Parietal⟶Acid
cells

**Body**

**Duodenum**

Chief⟶Pepsinogen
cells

**Pylorus**

**Antrum**

© Infobase Publishing

**Figure 2.5** Diagram of the stomach, and the substances produced by the different regions of the stomach.

joined to the jejunum, which is about 8 feet [2.5 meters] in
length. The jejunum is in turn joined to the ileum, which is
about 12 feet [around 3.6 meters] in length.

The small intestine is the site of most chemical (enzymatic)
digestion and the place from which the majority of nutrients are
absorbed in the body. When chyme reaches the small intestine,
it has been only partially digested by the stomach and duodenum. It is the small intestine's job to finish disassembly by taking up the digested nutrients and transporting them to the body.

The lining of the small intestine is an elaborate, ruffled structure with an enormous surface area that absorbs the nutrients
produced during the digestive process (Figure 2.6). As enzymes
break food into its molecular components, the nutrient-rich fluid
that is produced comes into contact with ruffled projections of
the intestinal lining (mucosa). These ruffles, called **villi** (singular
= **villus**), are finger-like extensions of the mucosal surface that
project into the **lumen**, or central cavity, of the intestine. Each

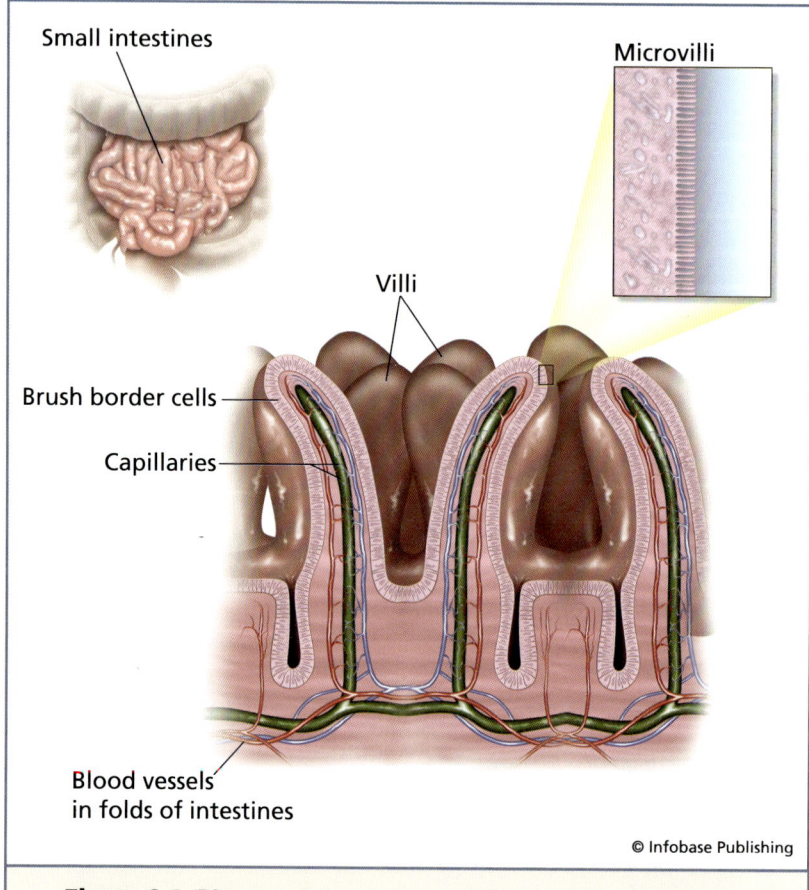

Small intestines

Microvilli

Villi

Brush border cells

Capillaries

Blood vessels
in folds of intestines

© Infobase Publishing

**Figure 2.6** Diagram of the structure of the small intestinal lining, illustrating the absorptive villi and microvilli, which together are responsible for the enormous absorptive capacity of this organ.

villus also contains thousands of microscopic projections called **microvilli** (singular = **microvillus**) that together create what is known as the **brush border** of the intestinal lining. Together, these structures increase the absorptive surface area of the small intestine by up to 600-fold, thereby greatly amplifying the capacity of the tissue to absorb nutrients. The absorptive surface area of the human small intestine has been estimated to be over 200 m$^2$, or about the size of a tennis court!

Once absorbed, the nutrients must also reach other cells and tissues that are not attached to the gastrointestinal tract. Each of the body's cells, from the brain to the toes, must be continually supplied with nutrients to function properly. To get transported around the body, these nutrients must enter the circulatory superhighway. To accomplish this, each microvillus contains a capillary that exports absorbed nutrients into the blood stream for delivery to the circulatory system.

Chyme is in constant motion in the small intestine due to the action of a series of muscular contractions. Muscle fibers that encircle the small intestine contract and relax rhythmically, churning the chyme and distributing it across the surface of the mucosa. This process repeatedly exposes the chyme to the small intestine's vast absorptive surface area. Other muscles that lie along the long axis of the intestine also contract and relax on alternating sides to slosh the chyme back and forth. Propulsive peristalsis also propels the chyme forward and moves it along the length of the small intestine like a conveyor belt, transporting it toward the large intestine.

What remains of the food that has passed through the small intestine is largely indigestible waste that must be expelled from the body; however, some nutrients and an appreciable amount of water still remain and must be absorbed by the colon, or large intestine. Thus, the major functions of the large intestine are absorption of water, salts, residual nutrients, and vitamins that are produced in the colon by intestinal bacteria, movement of indigestible waste material, and the formation of feces. Chyme is prepared for elimination by the activities of bacteria that reside in the colon. They ferment residual carbohydrates that were left undigested in the small intestine—releasing carbon, hydrogen and methane gas—and finish the breakdown of proteins. Bacteria also synthesize some substances required for normal metabolism, including vitamin K (needed for normal blood clotting) and certain B vitamins.

(*continued on page 36*)

## DIGESTION OF CARBOHYDRATES

Carbohydrates are the major source of energy for running the body's various chemical processes. This energy, stored in the chemical bonds of carbohydrate molecules, drives everything from metabolism to movement, enzyme activity, excretion, and growth. Carbohydrates are a large and diverse group of molecules composed chiefly of carbon, oxygen, and hydrogen. In addition to providing metabolic energy to the body, carbohydrates also form structural units. Deoxyribose, for example, is a sugar that makes up the backbone of DNA. The body can also convert carbohydrates into other compounds, such as fat (which is how calories from a candy bar find their way to our waistlines). Finally, carbohydrates can be converted into some amino acids to replenish proteins degraded by other metabolic processes.

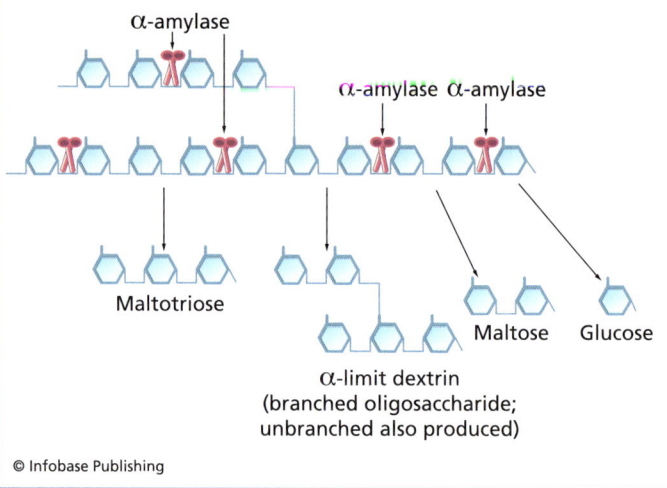

© Infobase Publishing

**Figure 2.7** Carbohydrate digestion illustrating the action of α-amylase in the breakdown of a complex carbohydrate. α-amylase enzymes cleave the chemical bonds between adjacent sugars in a starch molecule, releasing smaller, simpler sugars and oligosaccharides.

Carbohydrates can be divided into three major groups: monosaccharides (single-sugar molecules), disaccharides (a short chain of two sugar molecules), and polysaccharides (a chain of three or more sugar molecules). Monosaccharides and disaccharides are simple sugars. These include glucose, fructose (e.g., honey), and sucrose (table sugar). Reading any packaged food label will instantly reveal how common these items are in our everyday diet. Most mono and disaccharides are sweet, and hence large quantities are used in making desserts, sodas and candies.

Polysaccharides are the most complex type of carbohydrate. They are composed of long strings of monosaccharides, which can form either straight or branched structures. Polysaccharides usually lack the sweetness of the simpler sugars and many are not soluble in water. Vegetables, grains, and whole-grain breads contain an abundance of polysaccharides.

Examples of polysaccharides include glycogen, starch, and cellulose. Glycogen is a string of glucose that is made and stored in the muscles and liver, and used as an energy reserve. Starch is a major source of dietary carbohydrates (pasta, bread, and potatoes all contain an abundance of starch) and is digested in the mouth and intestine by the amylase enzymes (Figure 2.7). Starch is a plant product that is used by plants as an energy reserve, similar to the way glycogen is used by animals. When broken down by digestive enzymes, it is converted to glucose, which is why you may notice a sweet taste in your mouth after eating crackers or white bread. Because of its quick conversion to glucose, starch is used as a ready source of energy by animals.

Cellulose is also a product of plants. It is the major structural element of a plant's cell wall and is not digestible by humans. Cellulose is a major component of dietary fiber; it is thus often used as an ingredient in non-chemical laxative products.

(*continued from page 33*)

The colon is essentially a large reservoir of undigested food and bacteria. It lacks villi and microvilli, and therefore has a much smaller surface area for absorption. The colon can be conceptually divided into three segments: The ascending colon, the transverse colon and the descending colon (Figure 2.8). The ascending colon joins the small intestine at a junction called the **ileocecal valve**, which is essentially a one-way door that permits movement of food waste from the ileum into the colon but prevents backflow of material from the colon back to the ileum. The ascending colon then turns sharply to the left and becomes the transverse colon, which then turns again and becomes the descending colon. The descending colon joins the rectum at a juncture called the sigmoid colon (so-called because of its S-like shape). The rectum is the last stop for feces along the GI tract before they are eliminated from the body, pushed by powerful waves of the colon and rectum that propel the material out.

## THE PHYSIOLOGY OF DIGESTION: MECHANICS AND CHEMISTRY

Digestion actually begins with the brain. Close your eyes and imagine yourself eating your favorite meal. What do you feel? If you're like most people, your mouth begins to water and your stomach begins to rumble as you think about your first bite. These are the anticipatory reactions that your brain sets in motion to jump-start the process of digestion, and these occur before you even take your first bite.

Environmental signals prime the digestive process before food reaches the mouth. The sight, smell, or thought of food begins the flow of saliva and the secretion of stomach acid and enzymes, thereby preparing the digestive system to receive food. Saliva, an essential component of digestion, is produced by the salivary glands, located under the tongue near the lower part of the jaw. Not only does saliva lubricate food and facilitate chewing and swallowing, it also contains digestive

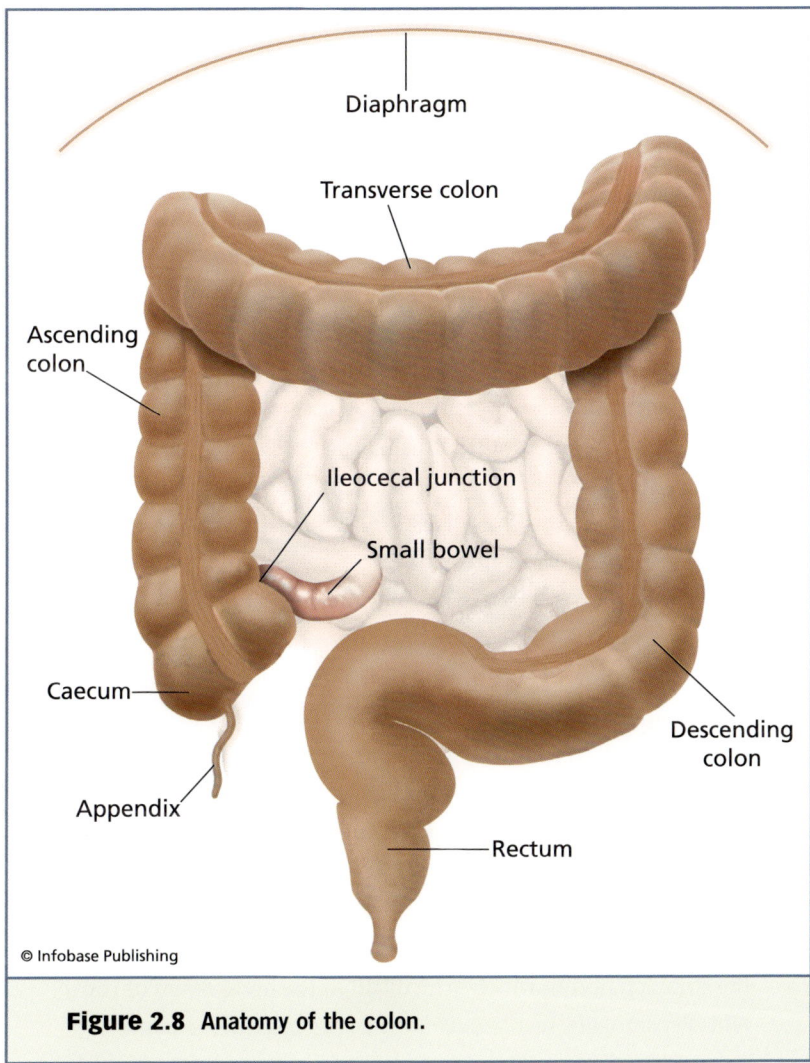

Figure 2.8 Anatomy of the colon.

enzymes, which are proteins that aid in the chemical breakdown of food.

As children, we're all taught to chew our food thoroughly.
This practice is not only good manners, it's also important for
digestion. Chewing grinds and shreds food, vastly increasing
the surface area upon which salivary enzymes can work in

breaking food down. These enzymes include **salivary amylase**—which begins the breakdown of carbohydrates—and **lingual lipase**—which aids the breakdown of fats. Thorough chewing also ensures that the food is well lubricated with saliva, making it easier to swallow.

The stomach is a large, muscular organ into which contents of the esophagus pass to undergo further processing. The stomach secretes a number of substances that aid in digestion, including hydrochloric acid and digestive enzymes. The stomach also agitates and churns food like a washing machine, mixing it with digestive acid and enzymes that, together, chemically break the food into small particles.

Cells in the lining of the stomach produce a number of substances that promote digestion. Upon stimulation by the brain and/or the arrival of food in the stomach, cells in the stomach begin to secrete hormones, acid, and enzymes. **G cells** (Figure 2.9), located near the bottom of the stomach, produce a hormone called **gastrin**. Gastrin is absorbed into the blood stream and carried to other secretory cells of the stomach, stimulating these cells to increase the production of stomach acid and digestive enzymes. Stomach acid is produced by a special type of cell located in the lining of the stomach's body called the **parietal cell**. This acid acts directly to break down food, but also acts indirectly by activating pepsinogen, an enzyme produced by **chief cells** (also located in the lining of the stomach body), which is involved in the breakdown of protein. Pepsinogen, secreted as an inactive enzyme, is converted to its active form, called **pepsin**, by exposure to stomach acid. Secretion of an inactive enzyme is a protective mechanism in the stomach, as its inactive nature protects the pepsinogen-producing cells from being digested by their own secretions. Chief cells, like all cells, contain protein and would be degraded

**Figure 2.9 (right)** Histology of the stomach illustrating the structures of each tissue region in the stomach and the cell types associated with the major functional region of the stomach.

## Gastric Glands

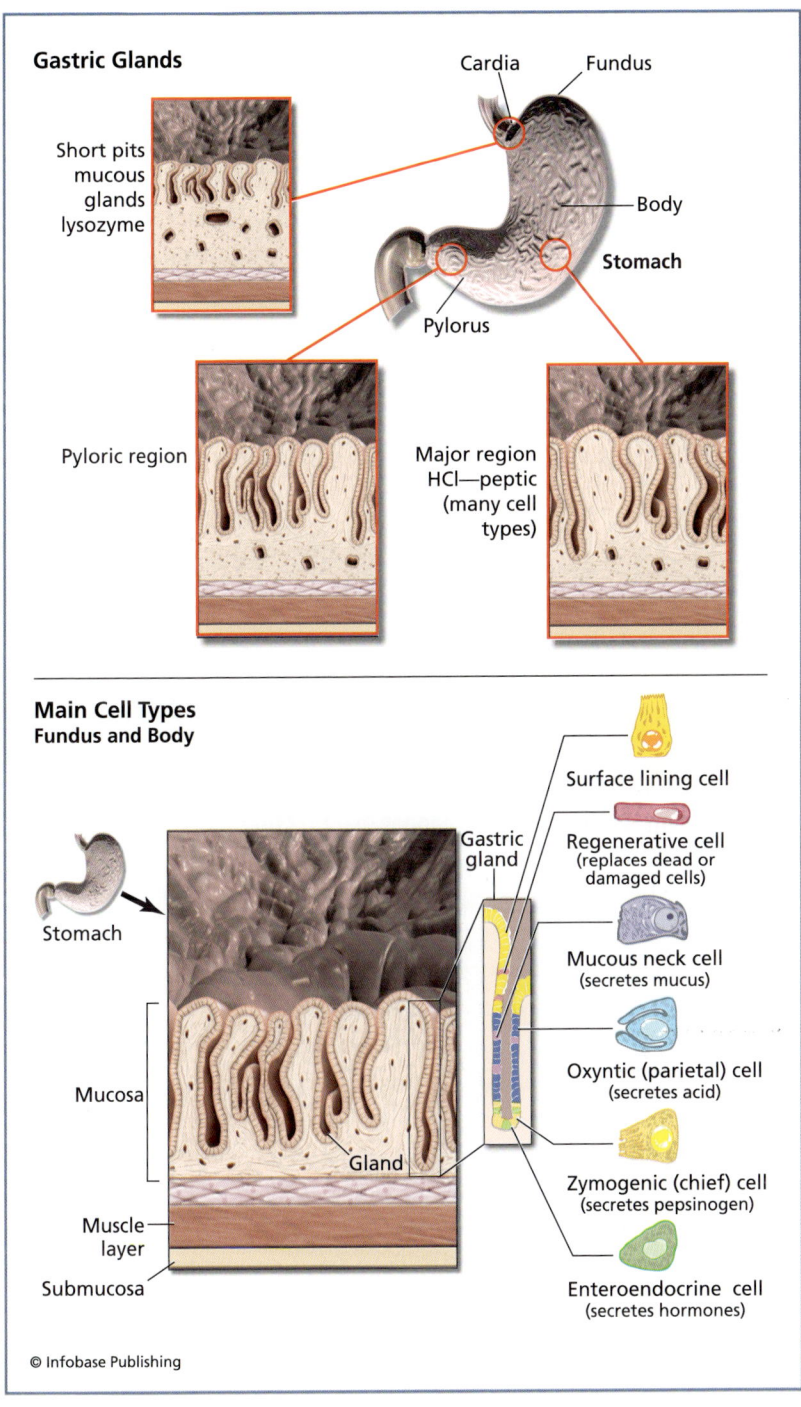

Cardia

Fundus

Short pits
mucous
glands
lysozyme

Body

**Stomach**

Pylorus

Pyloric region

Major region
HCl—peptic
(many cell
types)

## Main Cell Types
### Fundus and Body

Stomach

Gastric
gland

Surface lining cell

Regenerative cell
(replaces dead or
damaged cells)

Mucous neck cell
(secretes mucus)

Oxyntic (parietal) cell
(secretes acid)

Mucosa

Gland

Zymogenic (chief) cell
(secretes pepsinogen)

Muscle
layer

Submucosa

Enteroendocrine cell
(secretes hormones)

were pepsinogen produced as an active enzyme. The lining of the stomach itself is further protected by a thick layer of mucus, which is produced by **mucous cells** in the stomach lining. This mucus layer is often lacking in people who have ulcers. As we will see in later chapters, this reduction in mucus leads to auto-digestion of the stomach lining and the formation of ulcers, a phenomenon that occurs in people who are infected with *H. pylori*.

After food is sufficiently broken down by the churning and mixing with acid and enzymes, it flows into the duodenum. The duodenum regulates the flow of chyme from the stomach into the small intestine. It takes approximately two to six hours for the stomach to empty its contents into the duodenum. The

## DIGESTION OF FATS

Lipids, or fats, make up another group of nutrients essential to human function. Every cell is surrounded by a membrane composed mainly of lipids. Fats are also used as a chemical reservoir for energy storage. Although fat is manufactured in large amounts by the liver, not all fats can be made internally. Certain fats that the body cannot manufacture must be obtained in the diet. The body uses some of these essential dietary fats to make specific cellular structures (for example, sphingomyelin, which is used by brain cells), but dietary fat also aids in the absorption of fat-soluble vitamins from the intestines (such as vitamins A, E, and D).

Fats are chiefly composed of the same elements present in carbohydrates—carbon, hydrogen, and oxygen. But in fact these elements are present in different ratios and chemical configurations than they are in carbohydrates. A molecule of fat consists of two components: fatty acids and glycerol. One molecule of glycerol combines with three fatty acids to make up the structural unit of a fat. Most fats are insoluble in water, making them particularly challenging to digest since amount and composition of the chyme are both important in determining the rate of stomach emptying. High protein content and high acidity of the chyme slows stomach emptying, whereas low protein content and high volume promote emptying. High protein content triggers secretion of gastrin by cells in the duodenum, which reduces the rate of stomach emptying, affording high protein foods a longer stay in the bath of digestive enzymes.

The duodenum is also the receptacle for digestive enzymes produced by the pancreas, and for bile produced by the liver. The pancreas and liver are connected to the duodenum via a single tube-like structure called the **common bile duct**, through

the body is composed of over 70 percent water! Pancreatic and lingual lipase enzymes digest fat by breaking the fatty acids apart from the glycerol backbone, as illustrated in the diagram below (Figure 2.10).

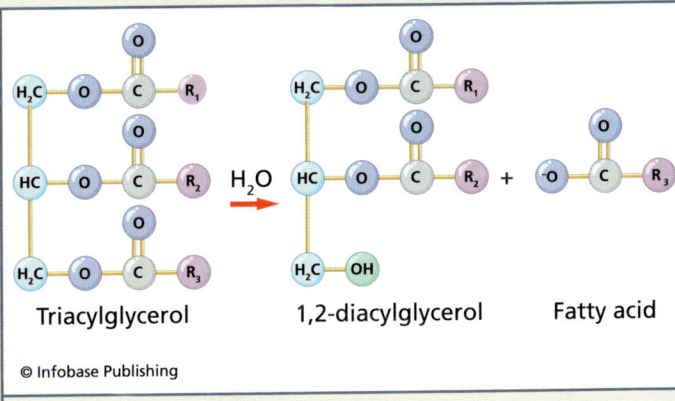

Triacylglycerol            1,2-diacylglycerol            Fatty acid

© Infobase Publishing

**Figure 2.10** Digestion of fat by breaking apart the fatty acids from the glycerol backbone.

which bile from the liver and gallbladder, and enzymes from the pancreas, flow. The pancreas produces numerous powerful digestive enzymes; however, because these enzymes are inactivated by acid, pancreatic enzymes are secreted in a highly alkaline liquid. This liquid rapidly neutralizes the highly acidic chyme, allowing the pancreatic enzymes to quickly digest the food.

The pancreas secretes enzymes that digest many types of foods. Pancreatic **proteases** such as **trypsin, chymotrypsin,** and **carboxypeptidase** digest proteins; pancreatic amylase is responsible for digestion of carbohydrates (sugars and starches) and **pancreatic lipase** digests **lipids** (fats and oils). These enzymes are similar to, but more potent than, the enzymes found in saliva: salivary amylase and lingual lipase.

Bile is a substance produced continuously by the cells of the liver and stored in the gallbladder. Bile performs a detergent-like function, acting somewhat like dish soap in a sink full of greasy dishwater. It emulsifies, or breaks, large globules of fat into smaller globules. By breaking the fat into small droplets, a greater surface area is exposed to digestive enzymes, thereby increasing the efficiency of fat digestion by the pancreatic lipase enzyme.

Once fully mixed with bile and digestive enzymes, chyme moves down the intestinal tract, where it is taken up by the microvillus cells of the small intestine and passed to the capillaries and into the bloodstream. The microvilli themselves also contain digestive enzymes on the surface of the cells that break down incompletely digested nutrients while the nutrients are being drawn into the tissue. On or adjacent to the cell membranes are enzymes that act on simple sugars to break them into individual sugar molecules; **peptidases**, which break down short fragments of proteins, called **peptides**, into individual amino acids; and lipases, which break down small fat molecules into their components: fatty acid and glycerol.

# 3

# H. pylori:
# Its Biology and Its
# Survival in the Stomach

Armed with a working knowledge of the digestive system, we can now look at how *H. pylori* infects people and sets up housekeeping in the human stomach. *Helicobacter pylori* is a rod-shaped, corkscrew-like bacterium that lives in the stomach and upper intestinal tract of infected people, and contributes to a variety of digestive system diseases. It has recently been identified as the primary cause of human **gastric** and **duodenal ulcers** (Figure 3.1).

## BACTERIAL CHARACTERISTICS OF *H. PYLORI*

*H. pylori*, like many pathogenic bacteria, is **Gram-negative**, a term that describes how the bacterium reacts with a particular type of stain. Gram staining is a technique used by medical laboratories to help identify bacteria when they are isolated from diseased tissue. The technique provides information about the outer membrane of the bacterium, which reveals much about its biology and potential for causing disease.

Unlike Gram-positive bacteria, Gram-negative bacteria contain an outer wall called the **lipopolysaccharide**, or LPS, layer. This serves as a protective layer through which materials must pass before they reach the cell. Gram-negative bacteria differ from one another in the composition of the LPS, particularly in the specific type of polysaccharide present in the membrane. In many Gram-negative species, this layer is toxic and responsible

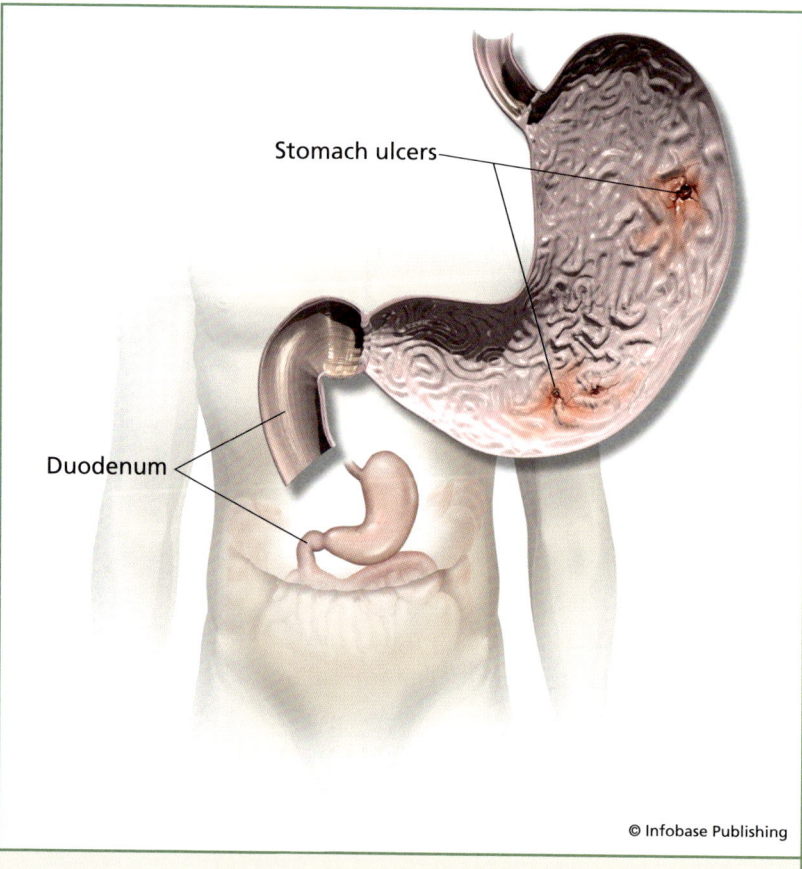

Stomach ulcers

Duodenum

© Infobase Publishing

**Figure 3.1** Illustration depicting appearance and location of gastric ulcers.

for some of the symptoms of an infection; hence components of the LPS layer are sometimes called **endotoxins**.

Beneath the LPS outer wall is a small, protective space called the **periplasmic space**, thought to be one way that *H. pylori* is able to survive in the stomach. Beneath that is a layer of **peptidoglycan**, a compound composed mostly of protein and polysaccharide, which is thicker in Gram-negative bacteria than Gram-positive species.

## *H. PYLORI'S* ADAPTATIONS TO ACIDITY

Despite the fact that *H. pylori* infection is one of the most common diseases on earth, its exact mode of transmission is not known. Because the organism lives in the stomach, the assumption is that *H. pylori* gets to the stomach via the mouth. However, the stomach isn't a terribly welcoming environment in which to live. It is essentially an acid bath filled with digestive enzymes, making it hard to imagine how any organism could manage to survive without being digested alive.

Indeed, though *H. pylori* inhabits the stomach, it has a clear preference for regions of low acidity, which explains the pattern of infection that is observed in diseased tissue. Under normal conditions, the **antrum**, a less acidic region of the stomach than the stomach body, is often the site of *H. pylori* colonization in infected people. Evidence of *H. pylori*'s dislike for acid is also supported by the following observation; when infected patients are given drugs that reduce acid production in the body of the stomach, the distribution of infection shifts toward that area. This suggests that under normal circumstances, the body of the stomach is too acidic for the organism to thrive. The observation that children, who have less stomach acidity than adults, are more easily infected further suggests that stomach acidity is indeed a barrier to *H. pylori* growth.

*H. pylori*'s intolerance of acid has led to its occupation of a unique niche in the body. Rather than living in the stomach's lumen, where acid concentrations are high, *H. pylori* lives deep in the mucus layer adjacent to the gastric mucosa. The mucus layer—a thick, **viscous** liquid composed of the glycoprotein **mucin**—effectively neutralizes the acid in the environment immediately adjacent to the stomach wall. This buffer protects the stomach tissue from its own acid secretions, and is therefore an extremely convenient habitat for a bacterium that cannot tolerate acid.

The difficulty for most organisms seeking to colonize this layer would be the viscosity of the mucin, which most bacteria

## GRAM STAIN

When a person walks into a doctor's office with an infection, how does the doctor know what type of infection the patient has? Typically the doctor will look at the infected tissue (the throat or a cut on the leg, for example), then take a swab of that tissue and send it to the lab for evaluation. The lab usually does several tests on the germs that they receive, but one of the first tests is the Gram stain.

The Gram stain was developed in 1884 by Danish bacteriologist Hans Christian Gram, who was looking for a method that would enable him to distinguish two different types of bacteria. This technique is still one of the most widely used methods in medical microbiology, and one of the quickest and easiest ways to categorize a bacterium obtained from an infected person. Not only does the Gram stain make it easy to see the size and shape of the bacteria under a microscope (it would otherwise be relatively transparent on a glass slide), it also tells the scientist a good deal about the materials that compose the bacterium's outer wall.

In the Gram staining procedure, a small amount of bacterium from a patient sample or, more often, from a culture is placed on a glass slide and allowed to dry. The slide is then heated briefly by passing it under a flame. The heating 'fixes' the bacterium to the glass slide to prevent it from washing off during the staining process. When the slide is cool, the sample

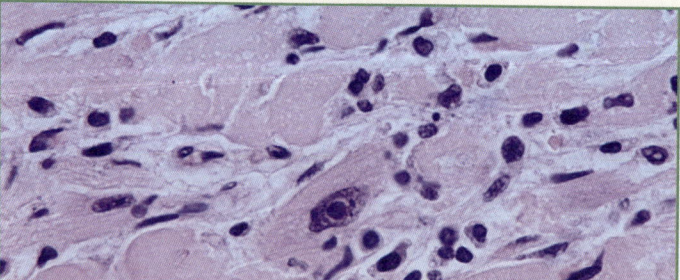

**Figure 3.2** This is a micrograph of Gram-positive bacteria. (CDC/Dr. Martin Hicklin)

is covered with a purple stain called Gentian Violet. After about a minute, the stain is washed off under running water and treated with Gram's solution, a mixture of water, iodine, and potassium iodide. After about 30 seconds, the Gram's solution is rinsed with ethyl alcohol and the slide is covered with another dye such as eosin or fuchsin (both of which are red).

Using this technique, Gram-positive bacteria are stained blue-black or purple by the combined action of the Gentian Violet and Gram's iodide solution, which react with one another and stain the inside of the cell (Figure 3.2 and 3.3). On the other hand, Gram-negative bacteria decolorize when washed with ethyl alcohol and become transparent, which is why the last step is to stain with a red dye that doesn't interfere with the Gram-positive bacterial stain and instead provides a red or pink tint to the Gram-negative bacteria. While it is not known why this staining procedure is effective, it is believed that the inner peptidoglycan layer of the Gram-negative bacteria is too thin to retain the stain inside of the bacterium. In Gram-positive strains, though, the peptidoglycan layer is thicker, helping to hold the stain in. The exact scientific reason for this difference is not known, yet the Gram stain is an extremely useful technique that helps doctors diagnose diseases in their patients.

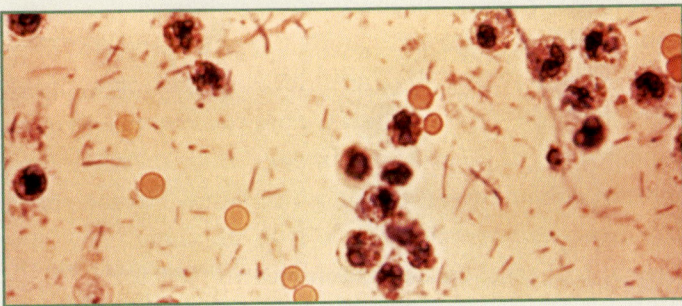

**Figure 3.3** This is a micrograph of Gram-negative bacteria. (CDC)

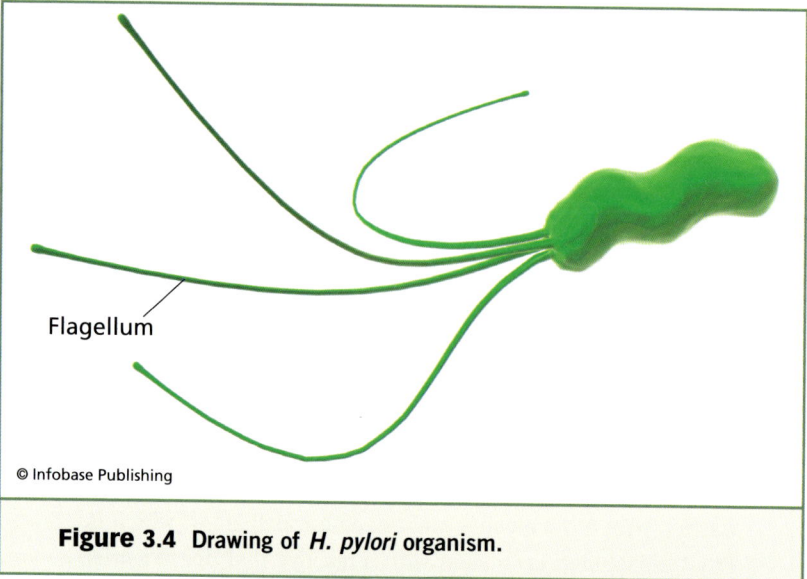

Flagellum

© Infobase Publishing

**Figure 3.4  Drawing of *H. pylori* organism.**

would be incapable of penetrating; however, *H. pylori* is equipped with a tuft of between four and seven whip-like structures (called flagella; singular = flagellum) (Figure 3.4) that beat back and forth, propelling it forward and allowing it to swim in liquid environments. This, combined with its corkscrew-like shape, allows *H. pylori* to burrow deeply into the mucus layer of the stomach, thereby escaping the acidity in the lumen. *H. pylori* also produces a protein that helps it penetrate the jelly-like layer of mucin. This protein, called **collagenase**, is believed to partially digest or liquefy the mucin, thereby reducing its viscosity and allowing the organism to move more freely (Figure 3.5).

 *H. pylori* is very efficient at locating and colonizing its intended target. This is perhaps because the swimming pattern exhibited by *H. pylori* is not random. *H. pylori* moves in a directed fashion toward mucin, which means that the organism possesses genes that enable it to somehow "sense" the chemicals of which mucin is composed and follow the chemical trail leading to the mucus layer (a sense that is somewhat akin to smelling).

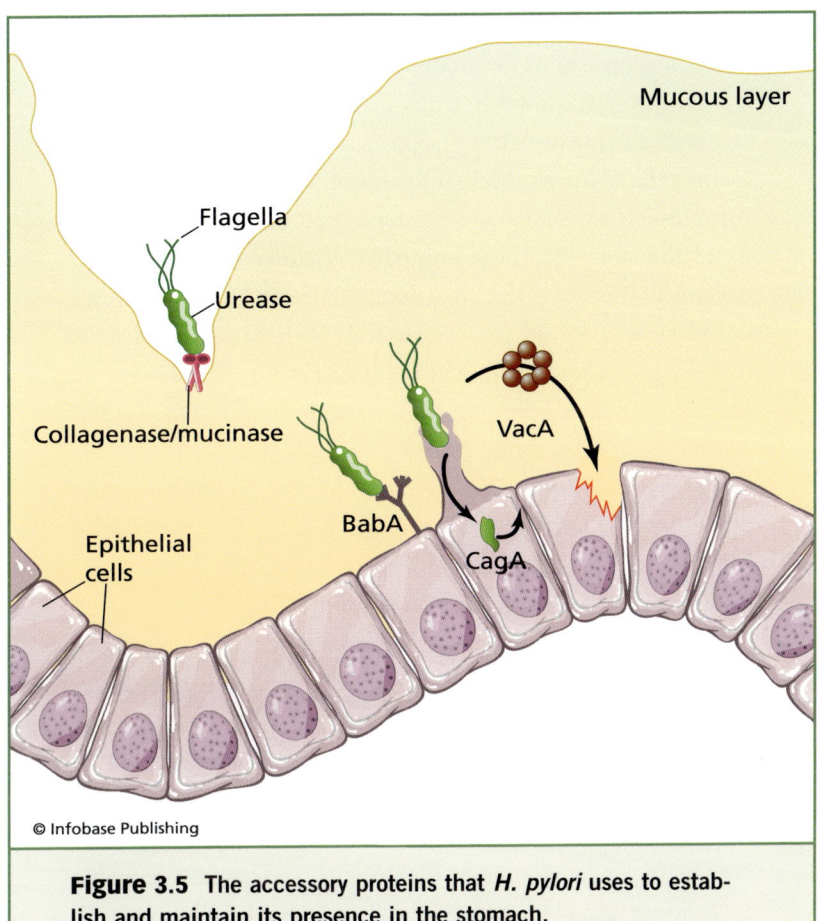

© Infobase Publishing

**Figure 3.5** The accessory proteins that *H. pylori* uses to establish and maintain its presence in the stomach.

No matter how quickly the bacterium swims, however, it must survive the stomach's acid at least temporarily to reach the mucin layer. *H. pylori* is a bacterium that prefers to grow at a neutral pH (that is, neither acidic nor basic). By altering the composition of its periplasmic space, it essentially forms a bubble around itself so that it can adapt to suit the requirements of its environment. Though the organism is not impenetrable to acid, altering the composition of this space provides a buffer zone between the outside world and its vital insides. In this way, *H. pylori* protects itself from being burned by the acid while in transit to its destination.

*H. pylori* accomplishes this feat in part by producing an enzyme called urease. Urease converts urea, a product secreted by the cells of the stomach, into ammonia and carbon dioxide. Ammonia is a weakly basic substance that neutralizes the acidity of the stomach in the immediate vicinity of the *H. pylori* organism. Because this reaction occurs in the organism's periplasmic space, *H. pylori* effectively bathes itself in an acid-buffering solution. As long as the bacterium is surrounded by this halo of ammonia as it moves through the stomach, it is relatively impervious to the stomach's acid.

*H. pylori* produces another enzyme, **alpha-carbonic anhydrase** ($\alpha$-CA), that also contributes to this de-acidification process. $\alpha$-CA cooperates with urease in the process of de-acidification by converting the carbon dioxide produced by urease into bicarbonate (a compound similar to baking soda). Bicarbonate is another weakly basic chemical that neutralizes the stomach's acidity.

The importance of these enzymes has been demonstrated by studies performed with experimental strains of *H. pylori* that lack either urease or $\alpha$-CA. Urease-negative strains are particularly inefficient at colonizing the stomach and have been unable to produce ulcers in experimental animals. In other experiments in which compounds that inhibit the urease enzyme were administered, the effect was the same: the bacterium was unable to colonize the stomachs of animals. Similarly, studies conducted with strains lacking $\alpha$-CA demonstrated that mutants were much less acid-tolerant than the strains containing $\alpha$-CA.

## HOW *H. PYLORI* STICKS TO YOUR STOMACH TISSUE

Getting settled is only the beginning, and many of the tricks that help *H. pylori* become established may also become necessary later in order to adapt to an ever-changing environment. For example, mucus is in constant turnover inside the stomach, and it is thought that the bacteria must repeat this colonization step, and burrow into newly formed mucus each time the mucus layer is shed from the stomach wall.

The peculiar thing is that *H. pylori*'s need for some, though not all, of these acid-adaptive measures decreases once the infection has become established, suggesting that maintenance of *H. pylori* infection is more complicated than once thought. Following colonization, for example, the need for urease diminishes, even though it continues to be made by the bacterium in large quantities. Evidence that urease expression is not related to infection maintenance or the resulting diseases was obtained using urease inhibitors on infected tissues. These studies revealed that once the mucus layer is colonized, chemicals that inhibit the activity of the urease enzyme do not cure the *H. pylori* infection, nor do they prevent ulcer formation, suggesting that the main function of the urease enzyme is to protect the bacterium until it colonizes the stomach's mucus layer. Whether this adaptive mechanism is turned on and off as the mucus layer is shed is not known.

Acid avoidance is only one method by which *H. pylori* retains its foothold in the stomach. Without some way to hold on to the tissue, the organism would be washed into the duodenum whenever the mucus layer is shed (a situation that undoubtedly occurs anyway in infected individuals, given that the duodenum is a major site of ulcer formation by *H. pylori*). To prevent detachment, *H. pylori* produces several types of adhesive proteins called **adhesins**. These proteins stick to specific lipids and carbohydrates that are normally present on the surface of the cells that line the stomach, preventing the organism from being dislodged by mechanical actions of the stomach (churning of food or the shedding of the mucus layer) (Figures 3.5 and 3.6). A large number of adhesin genes have been identified, and experimental strains in which these genes have been inactivated have demonstrated that the genes are essential to the survival of the bacterium.

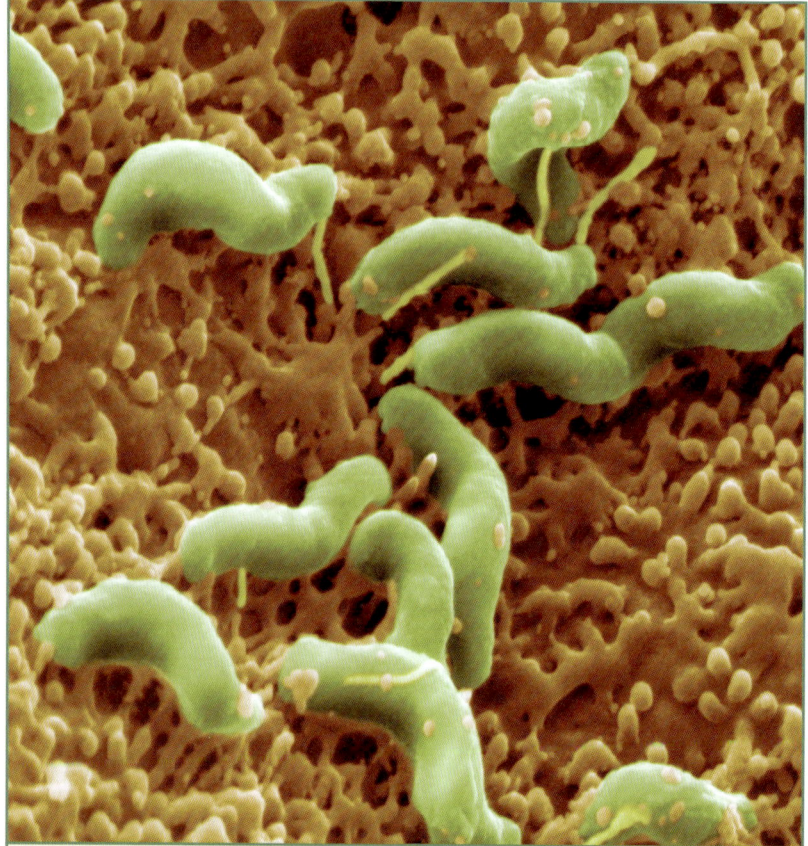

**Figure 3.6** *Helicobacter pylori* bacteria. (Eye of Science/Photo Researchers, Inc.)

Adhesin proteins are expressed on the outer membrane of the bacterium, functioning as anchors that fasten the organism onto the surface of the stomach. Their interaction with the molecules on stomach cells is somewhat like Velcro in that the two molecules (one on the surface of the bacterium and one on the mucosal cell of the stomach) stick to one another tightly by physically adhering to one another. These interactions are highly specific (like a lock and key); any given adhesin expressed on the *H. pylori* surface has affinity for only a specific molecule on the stomach cell's outer surface. For that reason, *H. pylori* cells express numerous different adhesins at the same time, meaning that each organism likely has multiple points of attachment with different types of molecules, making this a tight attachment, indeed.

However beneficial adhesins may be for *H. pylori*, some of these adhesins damage the lining of the stomach and lead to the pathology associated with infection. One adhesin, **BabA**, is particularly noteworthy because of its role in ulcer formation. BabA recognizes a polysaccharide-modified protein present on the surface of mucosal cells known as the **Lewis b antigen**. This antigen is present on a wide variety of cell types, particularly mucosal cells and blood cells. Attachment of *H. pylori* to the Lewis b antigen increases the body's immune response, which leads to the formation of antibodies against the stomach's own parietal cells (a type of **autoimmune response**); this damages stomach tissue and depletes the tissue of parietal cells.

It is noteworthy that not all strains of *H. pylori* express BabA protein. Strains that express BabA are associated with greater severity of disease than those that do not. This is presumably the result of the enhanced immune response in patients infected with BabA-expressing organisms, though this association has not been conclusively demonstrated. Therefore, while the immune response to infection is an essential bodily function, it can also contribute to the pathology of infectious diseases, particularly chronic infections, as will be discussed in later chapters.

# 4

# Who Is Infected with *H. pylori*?

Marlena is a 13-year-old patient from Peru. She lives in Lima, the country's capital, in a four-bedroom house with her parents, three grandparents, and six siblings. Compared with many families in Lima, hers is fairly well off. She is able to go to school, rather than having to go to work, and their house has indoor plumbing and hot water. However, her grandfather, who is 68 years old, recently developed severe stomach pains and was diagnosed with stomach cancer.

Because the doctors discovered that Marlena's grandfather was infected with *H. pylori*, they wanted to test her entire family. After a series of tests the doctors found that the entire family, even Marlena's two-year-old brother, was infected. Her father and grandmother, who have both had stomach pains for several years, were both found to have mild ulcers, but everyone else in the house seemed fine. Although she doesn't feel sick, the doctors insisted that Marlena take medicine to get rid of the infection, to make sure she doesn't develop an ulcer.

Marlena's mother was very upset. She prides herself on the cleanliness of her house and the health of her family. She was ashamed to find out that they had all become infected with a germ associated with poor sanitation, and she worried that she hadn't done enough to keep her family healthy; however, the doctor reassured her that it probably had nothing to do with her cooking or housekeeping. He said that over 60 percent of the people in Lima have the infection, and no one really knows where it comes from or how to prevent it. He also told her that she and her husband had most likely had the disease their whole lives, as most people in Peru become infected during childhood. He then gave the entire family advice about washing their food in sterilized water and boiling their drinking water, adding that periodic tests would be needed to ensure that the medicine eliminates the infection, and that frequent health checkups would be recommended to monitor for re-infection.

## MECHANISM OF INFECTION

Infection occurs when *H. pylori* is swallowed. Ingestion of the bacterium by consumption of contaminated food or liquid, or by eating unwashed vegetables contaminated with human sewage (as occurs often in developing countries), seems to be the most likely route of exposure; however, the bacterium has also been retrieved from vomit and dental plaques. There is also a great deal of evidence, obtained by studying infection patterns in populations, suggesting that *H. pylori* infects people via the mouth. And, as unappetizing as it sounds, the most likely route of exposure is via fecal-oral or oral-oral routes. Infection is highest in countries where sewage is not well contained or not adequately treated. The rate of infection is highest among families who have infected members, indicating that person-to-person contact is important. Indeed, in developing countries, it is often children who become infected. This may be the result of exposure by infected caregivers and siblings. Or it could reflect the fact that because children have less well-developed immune systems, they are less likely to resist an infection once exposed. In some countries, over 90 percent of the population is infected. So although the exact modes of transmission are not precisely known, it is apparent that the *H. pylori* colonizes the stomach rather effectively!

## UNDERSTANDING HOW
## *H. PYLORI* INFECTION SPREADS

Despite the fact that *H. pylori* infection is one of the most common infectious diseases on earth, the way in which it is transmitted is not precisely known. There are several reasons for this: First, there are numerous sources of infection. Second, people tend not to see their doctors when initially infected, so physicians are unable to precisely pinpoint where and how their patients became exposed. Finally, the symptoms, which are usually mild, are common to any number of other infections (such as the stomach flu). In fact, *H. pylori* infection is often diagnosed only when other diseases have been eliminated, a process that can take years.

Scientists have gotten around this mystery, at least somewhat, by studying the rate of infection in populations, hoping to find clues about what factors cause the infection to spread. These studies, called **epidemiologic studies**, are one way to study diseases before much is known about how they occur. **Epidemiologists**, who are scientists trained in the mathematical analysis of health data, work to determine causes of disease by examining data from large populations of people. They gather huge amounts of information from a wide array of sources and then perform mathematical analyses to determine whether there is any **statistical**, or mathematical, association between a given factor and the presence of the disease.

Epidemiologists make use of government health statistics, medical and death records, and personal interviews with patients and physicians to piece together the complex clues that tell the story of the disease-causing organism and its victims. They gather data about everything they can think of, such as the person's age, educational level, occupation, neighborhood, family size, diet, number and type of pets, marital status, and family medical history, to name a few. Then, by putting these clues together, the epidemiologist tries to identify things that infected people have in common, and how an infected person's lifestyle brings him or her into contact with the organism. Individually, factors like age, gender, or income seem very general and do not reveal much about the disease, but when placed together a pattern begins to emerge.

## SOURCES OF INFECTION

After innumerable epidemiologic studies of *H. pylori* infection patterns worldwide, one factor emerges as the most important determinant of infection: poverty. Does this mean that everyone who has an *H. pylori* infection is poor, or that all poor people are infected? Definitely not.

So how does poverty cause *H. pylori* infection? It doesn't, actually, but as you will see from the discussion that follows, impoverished communities have characteristics that may facilitate the spread of the *H. pylori* infection from person to person. These factors, which include overcrowding, poor sanitation, insects, lack of adequate facilities with which to boil water or thoroughly cook food, and consumption of contaminated produce, allow the organism to travel easily from person to person.

### Person-to-Person Contact

Benin is a country in sub-Saharan, western Africa, situated between Nigeria and Togo; over 75 percent of its population is infected with *H. pylori.* It is a hot, humid country that is home to over five million people, some in very crowded and unique settings. One village in Benin is in the middle of a large, shallow lake containing numerous small, thatch-roof huts built on stilts that house large, extended families in very close quarters. Other villages, built on dry land, consist of numerous small, mud huts that house large families of parents, children, and grandparents, as well as aunts, uncles, and cousins. Families in Benin live in close contact, and modern sanitary devices, such as flush toilets, are at a minimum.

Epidemiologists studying the transmission of *H. pylori* have found that infection tends to run in families, and that living in the city poses more of a risk than living in the country. This suggests that overcrowding is one factor that promotes the spread of the disease. In fact, the research has shown that the more crowded a person's home, the more likely he or she is to be

## STATISTICS AND EPIDEMIOLOGY

A statistical association is one in which, mathematically speaking, two (or more) things occur more often together than they do apart. This association is called a correlation.

The two graphs (Figure 4.1) mathematically illustrate the concept of a correlation. The top graph shows an example of a perfect positive correlation between two variables, X and Y. In this example, Y varies as a function of X, so that any change in X is reflected by an equal change in Y. Thus, it might be assumed that X and Y are interdependent, or, in other words, Y is dependent on X. On the other hand, the graph on the bottom illustrates an example of two variables that are not statistically correlated. In this case, whatever value X takes, Y is always the same. In other words, the factor X has no effect on factor Y.

This concept of correlation is used to understand cause and effect. For example, there is a correlation between rain and the presence of clouds in the sky and between cigarette smoking and lung cancer. The correlation between rain and clouds or between cigarette smoking and lung cancer implies (but does not prove) that there is some kind of relationship between those pairs of variables that scientists can further investigate.

Sometimes, however, correlations derived from statistical analyses of data lead to complicated associations that are much more difficult to interpret. For example, an epidemiologist may find an association between a person's educational level and a particular kind of disease (such as lung cancer). At first, that association might not prove to be very helpful in identifying the specific cause of the disease, but it might help the scientist narrow the search for causes.

For example, if the majority of people in a particular population who develop lung cancer never went to college, one might assume that there was something about having gone to college that prevents a person from developing lung cancer. The next step would be to figure out what it was about college-educated people that was different from people who never went to college. By interviewing a number of people who went to college and a number who didn't, the scientist might find that fewer people in the college-educated group smoked cigarettes compared to the no-college group, and this might help the scientist identify the true cause of the association (in this case, between smoking and cancer).

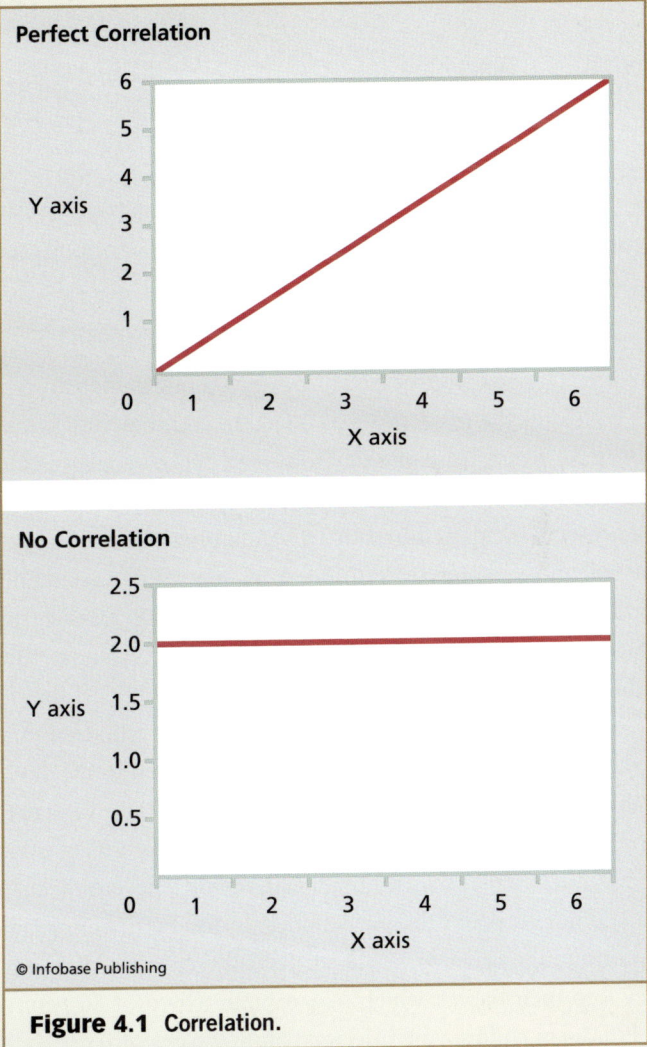

**Figure 4.1**  Correlation.

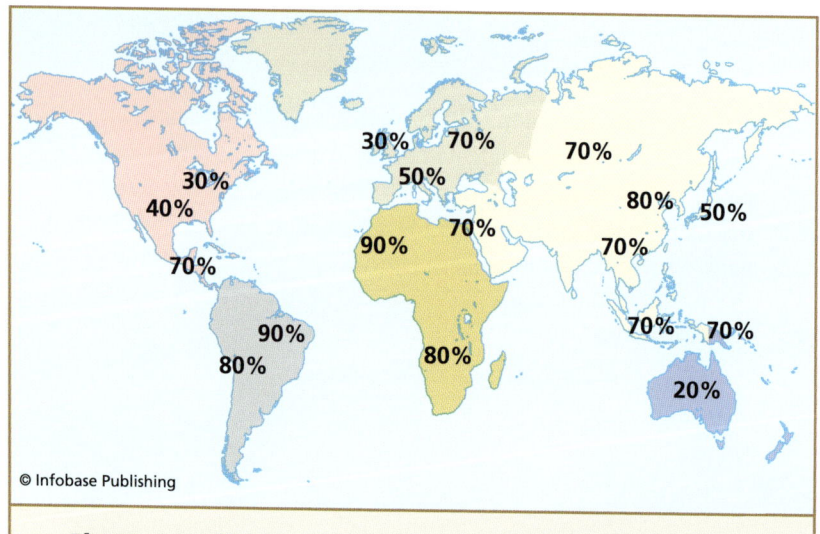

**Figure 4.2** This map of the world shows the percentages of *H. pylori* infection.

infected. This key piece of evidence suggests that person-to-person contact is the main route of infection and that, rather than getting *H. pylori* from the environment, most people tend to become infected by other members in their households. Upon examination of all members of a given family, it became apparent that most people were infected in infancy or early childhood, and that the risk was greatest when the mother was infected, implying that parents transmit the bacterium to their children.

Several things that mothers do for their children may explain this high rate of infection among children in the developing world (Figure 4.2). In India, where mothers moisten their nipples with saliva before feeding their infants, the rate of infection is much higher than among neighboring Pakistani women, who do not. Also, in Ethiopia, where baby food is not affordable or commonly available, mothers partially chew the food that they feed their babies, which may explain why over 80 percent of Ethiopian children are infected before the age of six.

## Poor Sanitation and Contaminated Food

While person-to-person contact is thought to be the most likely cause of infection, other factors are undoubtedly at work. Fecal-oral exposure is one route by which many people become infected with *H. pylori*. Because *H. pylori* is shed in the feces of infected persons, poor sanitation leads to increased exposure. This is particularly true in impoverished agricultural areas where soil is fertilized with human sewage. Growing food in fecally-contaminated soil may lead to increased rates of infection, particularly when the food is either poorly cooked or uncooked (such as salad vegetables).

## Drinking Water

In addition to person-to-person contact, other sources of infection have been identified. In Peru, a country with very high rates of *H. pylori* infection, contaminated drinking water was found to be one source of transmission. In one study, more people who drank water from their city's water supply were infected than those who used well water. Further studies in Peru demonstrated that *H. pylori* was indeed present in the drinking water, and that people who boiled their water had lower rates of infection than those who did not. This suggests that *H. pylori* infection can also be spread through drinking water, particularly in countries in which water sanitation is poor and drinking water is not sanitized in the home by boiling or chlorination.

## Insects

Insects may be another source of food contamination. Houseflies have been repeatedly implicated as agents in the spread of *H. pylori*. The bacterium can live for up to 12 hours on the body of a housefly, and for more than 24 hours in its intestine. As flies move across food or other surfaces, they leave droppings that contain bacteria, which can then be ingested and lead to infection. Along a similar vein, feces of cockroaches that have been fed *H. pylori* cultures can be found to contain the bacterium for up to 24 hours, suggesting that food contaminated with the fecal material of these insects can transmit the bacterium to humans, particularly if the food is not properly cooked or washed with clean water.

## DEVELOPED COUNTRIES

The pattern of infection in developed countries differs markedly from that of developing countries, and the underlying causes of infection in developed countries are less clearly defined. In the US, Canada, and Western Europe the rate of infection is comparably quite low. The frequency of infection in these countries increases with age, suggesting that the most common mode of transmission is probably not parent to child. The practice of water chlorination and the widespread availability of flush toilets and sewage disposal systems reduce the opportunity for infection in the general environment.

While the overall rate of infection is lower in developed countries, it is not uniformly lower. There are pockets of infection in developed countries, some of which are associated with poverty, the strongest factor determining the pattern of infection. Also, immigrant populations whose origins are in developing countries typically have higher rates of infection than the general population. For example, in a recent study of *H. pylori* infection rates of Mexican-Americans, the rate of infection among recent Mexican immigrants was similar to the rate of infection in Mexico, but among Mexican-Americans born in the U.S., the rate of infection was more similar to the U.S. population-at-large.

## THE ROAD AHEAD: WHAT EPIDEMIOLOGY HAS TAUGHT US

Epidemiological studies on *H. pylori* transmission have told us something about which infection management strategies

**Table 4.1** *H. pylori* Adult Infection Rate from selected countries.

| | Country | Adult Infection Rate (%) |
|---|---|---|
| **Africa** | Algeria | 43–92 |
| | Ethiopia | >95 |
| | Gambia | >95 |
| | Kenya | 94 |
| | Nigeria | 69–91 |
| | Zaire | 77 |
| **Asia** | Bangladesh | 75–90 |
| | China | 86 |
| | India | 77–88 |
| | Papua New Guinea | 36–75 |
| | Saudi Arabia | 40–70 |
| | Siberia | 85 |
| | Sri Lanka | 72 |
| | Thailand | 74 |
| | Australia | 30.6 |
| **Central America** | Guatemala | 58–65 |
| | Mexico | 60 |
| **Europe** | Finland | 34 |
| | Italy | >40 |
| | San Marino | 51 |
| | Spain | 50–80 |
| | Greenland | 58 |
| **Middle East** | Egypt | 90 |
| | Jordan | 82 |
| | Libya | 75–94 |
| | Saudi Arabia | 80 |
| | Turkey | 80–100 |
| | New Zealand | 4.1–6.6 |
| **North America** | United States | 35–40 |
| | Canada | 20–40 |
| **South America** | Argentina | 38–62 |
| | Bolivia | 81 |
| | Brazil | 82 |
| | Chile | 72 |
| | Colombia | 54–68 |
| | Costa Rica | 68 |
| | Peru | 60–92 |

are likely to be most effective; specifically, strategies addressing the fundamental issues of poverty are likely to be the most successful. These studies have also shown that providing access to clean water, containment of sewage, and educating parents about the best ways to avoid the spread of *H. pylori* to their children will help to reduce the number of new cases each year; however, this will be a long and difficult road. Resources that are needed to build the kind of infrastructure required for water treatment and sewage containment are simply unavailable throughout most of the world.

Furthermore, traditions and cultural practices strongly influence the ways in which people relate to one another, and thus changes affecting interactions between family members may be difficult to implement. There are also practical limitations to how much a society can adapt, given the resources available to it. For example, in countries where food supplies are limited, it will be difficult for mothers to avoid pre-chewing the food that they feed their babies.

Each country will undoubtedly have to develop solutions that conform to its cultural values and available resources. By virtue of its enormity alone, the problem of *H. pylori* infection will have no simple solutions. Working to improve living conditions in impoverished countries and providing education about the disease and its spread will be the best places to start, a process that will necessitate greater international investment if the spread of this disease is to be slowed.

# 5

# *H. pylori* and Ulcers

**If you set out to build a super-successful microorganism, how would you do it?** First, you might ask what makes a microorganism successful? Most biologists would argue that a successful microorganism avoids being killed and therefore reproduces well and spreads widely. So, if your microorganism had an animal host, would it be better to maim and kill the host, or live quietly without causing trouble and thereby escape notice?

Bacteria have caused many of humankind's most dreaded illnesses (the plague, typhoid fever, cholera, botulism, and tetanus, to name a few). Although the names of these diseases might be household words, it could be argued that the bacteria that caused them are not particularly successful. Because they cause severe illness and/or death, they do not have an opportunity to spread widely before the host dies or becomes too ill to effectively pass the germ along. This is not the case with *Helicobacter pylori*.

The fact that *H. pylori* lives quietly inside the human stomach is what makes it such a successful organism. In most people there are no symptoms of infection, while in others the symptoms are mild. Only a tiny percentage exhibit symptoms noticeable enough that the person seeks medical care, and this often occurs decades after the initial infection, leaving plenty of time to infect others along the way. Typically, the symptom that brings patients to the doctor is an intense, gnawing or burning pain in the stomach, which signals the formation of an ulcer.

Ulcers were once thought to be caused by emotional stress and lifestyle (alcohol, smoking, etc.), but it is now recognized that the majority of them are the result of *H. pylori* infection. *H. pylori* infects over half the world's population, but only about 10 percent of the population develop ulcers. This discrepancy has puzzled investigators for decades.

Why do only certain people exhibit symptoms of *H. pylori* infection? Is it some property of the individual, or something about the organism that makes the disease worse in some individuals than others? The answer is probably both. Individual differences in how the host's immune system responds to infection combined with the nature of the infecting strain (i.e., what genes it carries) conspire to create greater damage in some people than in others. The diseases that *H. pylori* causes are thought to arise as a result of both direct damage by the bacterium and injury brought about by the host's own immune system.

## PATHOGENIC MECHANISMS: BACTERIAL GENES AND HOST IMMUNITY

When *H. pylori* infects the stomach or duodenum, it does a number of things to become established in the tissue. It must penetrate the mucus layer, attach to the surface of the epithelial cell, and acquire nutrients in order to survive. Several genes that help the organism perform those important functions also lead to damage of the host's stomach (Figure 5.1).

For example, the bacterial urease enzyme, which protects the organism from stomach acid, leads to the production of ammonia at the surface of the stomach or duodenum. Ammonia is toxic to cells and causes direct damage to the mucosal epithelial cell layer.

Once *H. pylori* attaches to the mucosal cells the organism manufactures other products that have more serious consequences for the tissue. In some, but not all, strains of *H. pylori*, a protein called **CagA** (cytotoxin associated gene A) is expressed. Strains that express this protein are strongly associated with the development of diseases such as ulcers and stomach cancer. The bacterium makes this protein and physically injects it into the mucosal cells using a syringe-like bacterial structure called the **pilus** (Figure 5.2).

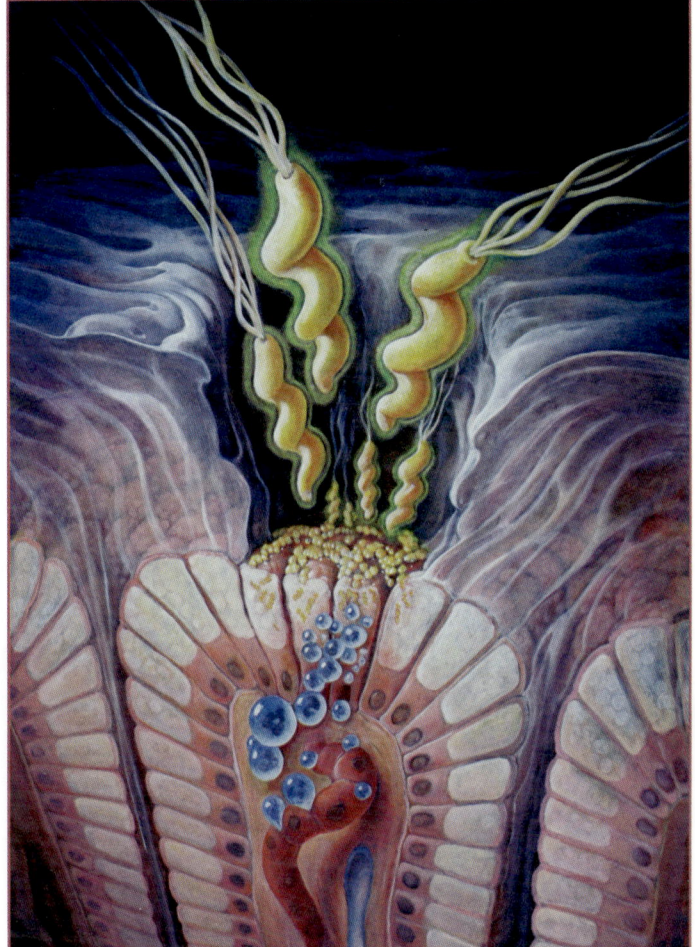

**Figure 5.1** *Helicobacter pylori* creating a stomach ulcer. (Carl Donner/PhototakeUSA.com)

Once inside the cell, CagA damages the epithelium by dismantling the structures that hold neighboring cells together. These points of attachment are known as **tight junctions**, which are impermeable barriers that prevent the free flow of large molecules (such as proteins and polysaccharides) between the lumen of the stomach and the deeper tissue layers

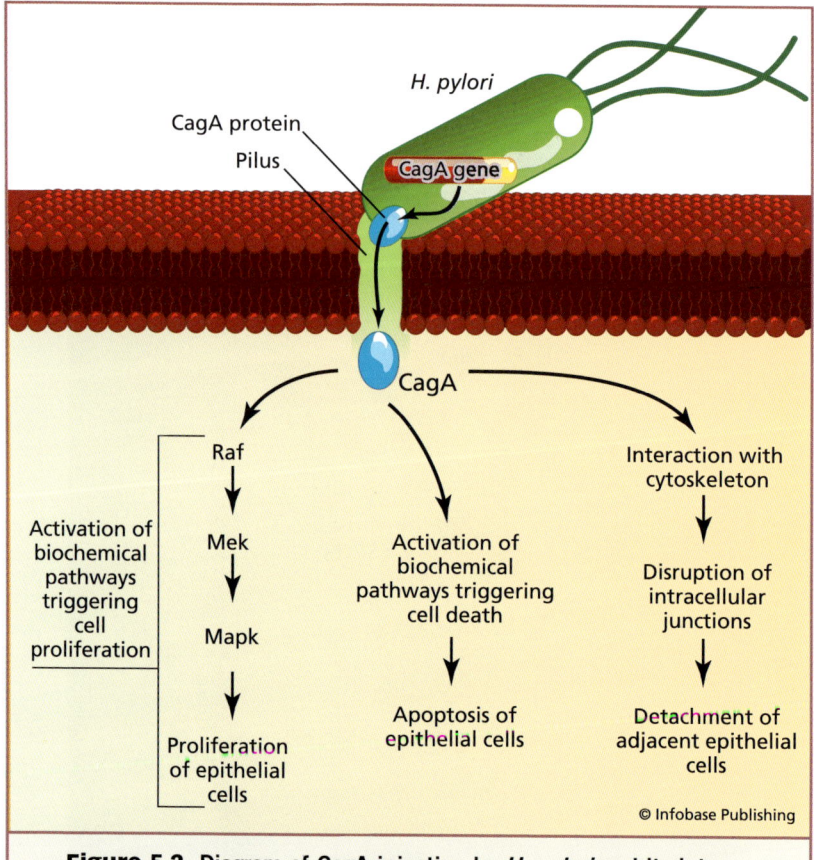

CagA protein
Pilus
H. pylori
CagA gene
CagA

Activation of biochemical pathways triggering cell proliferation

Raf
↓
Mek
↓
Mapk
↓
Proliferation of epithelial cells

Activation of biochemical pathways triggering cell death
↓
Apoptosis of epithelial cells

Interaction with cytoskeleton
↓
Disruption of intracellular junctions
↓
Detachment of adjacent epithelial cells

© Infobase Publishing

**Figure 5.2** Diagram of CagA injection by *H. pylori* and its interaction with the host cells and proteins.

below. By unlocking the tight junctions, *H. pylori* obtains nutrients such as proteins and polysaccharides that it needs for growth and survival. However this is destructive to the architecture of the tissue, damaging the protective layer of the tissue.

Another product associated with the formation of ulcers that *H. pylori* makes is the protein **VacA** (see Figure 3.5). Like CagA, this protein is a mechanism by which *H. pylori* can gain access to nutrients that would otherwise be unavailable. VacA is released outside the bacterium and then binds to the outer membrane of a stomach cell and either forms pores through which nutrients may leak, or induces the formation of large membrane-enclosed, bubble-like structures called **vacuoles** inside the cell (Figure 5.3). These vacuoles may also contain a number of substances useful to the bacterium, such as protein, polysaccharides, ions, and salts. VacA can also form vacuoles inside other membrane-enclosed structures of the mucosal cell. One such structure, the **mitochondrion**, is responsible for manufacturing most of the energy that the cell needs to survive. VacA protein inserts itself into the mitochondrial membrane, causing the mitochondrion to spill its contents, thereby killing the cell.

All of this cellular destruction alerts the immune system to the fact that there is something going on in the interior of the stomach. Chemical messengers, called **cytokines**, produced by sick and injured cells, send signals to the cells of the immune system, leading to an infiltration of immune cells into the tissue. This tissue becomes **inflamed**, a term used to describe the redness, swelling, and accumulation of immune cells that occurs at the site of infection.

Pathologists refer to the condition as **gastritis**, a well-known risk factor in the formation of ulcers. The cells of the immune system unleash very powerful chemical weapons to fight the invading bacteria; however, in the fight there is an appreciable amount of damage to the mucosal epithelial cells themselves.

Despite all the efforts of the immune system, the bacterial infection is often not cleared. This sets up cycles of repeated colonization and inflammation that result in loss of cells from the lining. The result is in a condition known as **gastric atrophy**, which is accompanied by a reduction of the protective mucus layer. The diminished amount of mucus is caused, at least in part, by the destruction of the cells that produce it. What results is a weakened area in the protective mucosal epithelial layer that allows stomach acid and digestive enzymes to get through to the lining beneath the epithelial cells. The acid and enzymes irritate and degrade the supportive lining beneath the mucosal epithelial layer and cause an open sore to form: an ulcer.

## PEPTIC AND DUODENAL ULCERS

Sores of this nature can occur in either the stomach or the duodenum. These sores can become very deep indeed, and the damage may become so severe that it eats through the entire thickness of the organ's wall. This is known as a **perforated ulcer** and is considered a medical emergency. Patients who have perforated ulcers may or may not have severe pain, but the outcome of a perforated ulcer is that, ultimately, bacteria, chyme, stomach acid, and digestive enzymes can leak into the abdominal cavity, creating a widely disseminated infection known as **peritonitis**, or inflammation of the membrane that covers the organs and abdominal cavity.

Ulcers can also form in the vicinity of blood vessels that supply the walls of the stomach or duodenum, and, if severe enough, can lead to damage of the vessel wall and leakage of blood into the ulcerated tissue. This is known as a bleeding ulcer. The main symptom of a bleeding ulcer is dark, tarry stool. This happens because the blood that leaks into the digestive system is digested along with food, and the breakdown of blood releases **hemoglobin** (the red pigment in blood cells that carries oxygen). The iron-containing hemoglobin adds a dark pigment to the stool.

If the bleeding is severe enough, anemia can result. Anemia is a reduction in the mass of red blood cells in the circulation, which can occur if a large amount of blood is lost from the ulcerated vessel. The symptoms of anemia include fatigue, pale skin and gums, and dizziness.

## OTHER CAUSES OF ULCERS

If you've read some of the other chapters closely, you may remember that approximately 90 percent of ulcers are caused by *H. pylori.* If you remember that number, you may be asking, "What causes the other 10 percent?" The most common cause of ulcers, other than *H. pylori,* is frequent, long-term use of nonsteroidal anti-inflammatory drugs (NSAIDs). These drugs, which include such household names as ibuprofen (brand names include Advil or Motrin), naproxen (also sold under the brand name Aleve), or aspirin (brand name Bayer or Ecotrin), can irritate and erode the lining of the stomach, leading to an acid- and digestive enzyme-induced destruction of the stomach lining resembling that caused by *H. pylori.* Many prescription versions of these drugs can also injure the stomach lining. Prescription NSAIDs such as celecoxib (Celebrex), valdecoxib (Bextra), meloxicam (Mobic), and naproxen (Naprosyn) can also cause a similar injury to the stomach.

# 6

# *H. pylori* and the Immune System

The immune system is a double-edged sword. Although well adapted for fighting infections, it also inflicts its own type of damage on normal tissue. The cells of the immune system are trained killers, but like bombs in a war, their killing mechanisms are somewhat indiscriminate. The inflammatory response that occurs in response to infection with *H. pylori* is both helpful and detrimental to the stomach tissue, as will be described below.

## INFLAMMATION AND IMMUNITY

The primary reaction of the immune system to *H. pylori* is inflammation. Inflammation is a complicated set of cellular and chemical responses occurring in infected or injured tissue. Infections (viral, bacterial, or fungal), trauma, or physical or chemical burns are all capable of eliciting an inflammatory response. The hallmark symptoms of inflammation are redness, heat, swelling, and pain at the site of injury. Large inflammatory responses, like those occurring during a case of pneumonia, have systemic effects outside the infected organ. These might include symptoms such as fever, chills, loss of appetite, and fatigue. The initial immune response to a bacterial infection is performed by the innate immune system, a collection of cells and chemical processes that together respond immediately to a threat. However, the innate immune system is not specific to the organism it is fighting, and thus is fairly indiscriminate in its actions—the mission of the innate immune system is simply to kill, and this can often be at the expense of other neighboring cells.

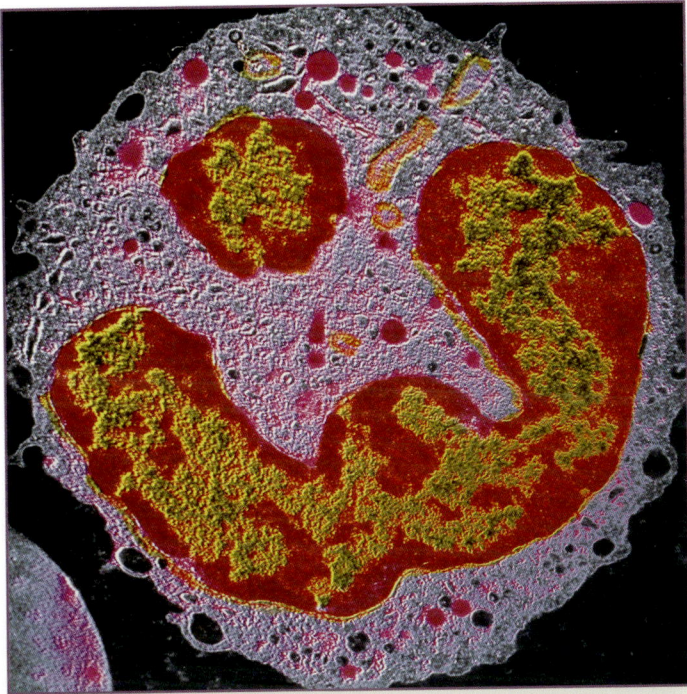

**Figure 6.1** This is a false-color transmission electron micrograph (TEM) of a single neutrophil, the most common type of white blood cell. (CNRI/Photo Researchers, Inc.)

The first step in the **innate immune process** is the recognition that a microbe invasion is underway. White blood cells become alerted to the presence of the invading microbes via chemical signals emitted by other cells, or by "sensing" the presence of the microbe through the chemicals the invading organism itself releases (such as endotoxin). Often the first cells to get the message that an invasion is underway are white blood cells called **neutrophils** (Figure 6.1). Neutrophils that are passing through blood vessels adjacent to the damaged tissue become sticky in response to the chemical signals coming from infected or injured tissues (Figure 6.2). This stickiness is due to proteins

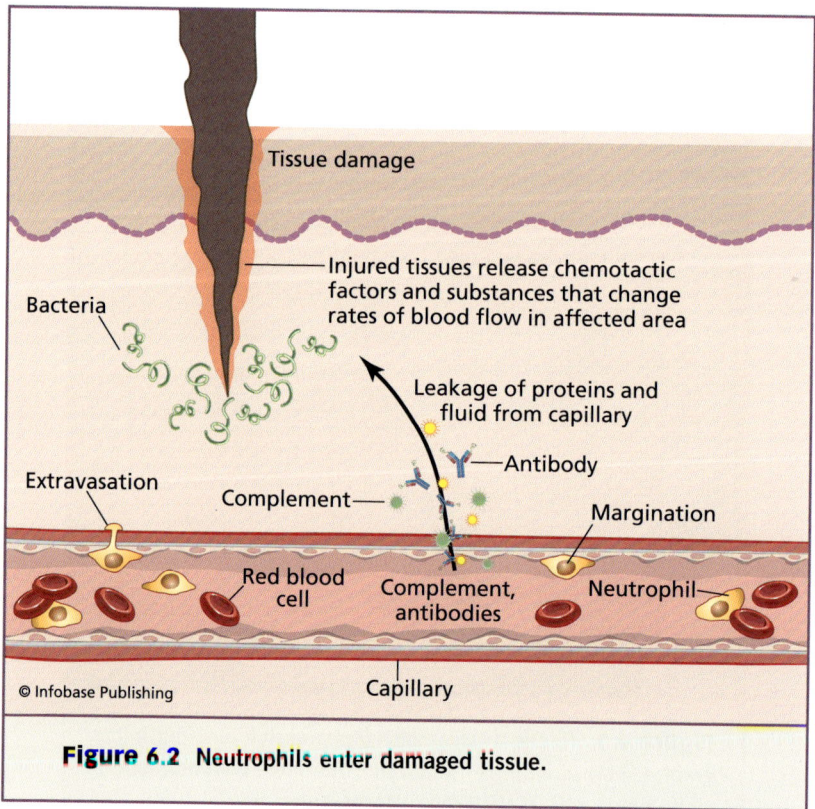

Figure 6.2 Neutrophils enter damaged tissue.

and polysaccharides on the outside of the neutrophil's cell membrane that respond to the presence of the chemical distress signals emitted by the tissue. Sticky neutrophils adhere to the walls of the blood vessels and migrate out of the blood by squeezing between the cells that line the wall of the vessel, and then enter the tissue. (Figure 6.2) The process by which they crawl through the spaces between the cells lining the vessels is called **extravasation**.

Once out of the vessel, the neutrophils follow the chemical trail produced by the damaged tissue or the invading bacteria. The process by which cells migrate in response to a chemical signal or chemical attractant is known as **chemotaxis**. Similar to a bloodhound following the trail of its quarry, chemotactic cells follow the chemical "scent" that leads them to where the action is. A number of chemicals can serve as chemotactic attractants, including bacterial products, cell and tissue debris, and a blood protein known as **complement**.

Complement is made by the liver and certain immune cells, and has a strong affinity for bacterial cell walls. It becomes activated by the presence of bacterial products, and sticks all over the outside of the bacterium in a process called **opsoniza-tion**. Opsonized bacteria behave, chemically speaking, like big flashing lights to chemotactic white blood cells, drawing the cells to their targets. White blood cells have proteins on their surfaces that recognize the complement that is adhered to the bacteria, and this helps the white blood cell stick to its target and eliminate it. Complement activation also initiates a very complex series of chemical reactions that greatly amplify the immune response, thereby drawing in additional cells from the blood.

One type of white blood cell recruited by this inflamma-tory response is the **macrophage**. Macrophages can arrive from the circulation via the blood vessels, or they can be resident in the tissue and recruited to the site of infection by the action of the neutrophils, or by the actions of the bacteria themselves. Macrophages, like neutrophils, are the cells that arrive early during an immune response, and they are the housekeepers that help clean up the infection. Like neutrophils, macrophages also respond chemotactically to activated complement and are attracted to opsonized bacteria.

Once the macrophages arrive at the site of infection, they produce additional chemical stimulants, known as **cytokines**, which do a variety of things to amplify the immune response. Inflammatory cytokines increase localized blood flow in the area of the infection (causing redness) and increase the perme-ability of the blood vessels. This increased blood flow brings additional white blood cells to the tissue and increases the tem-perature of the inflamed tissue (causing the sensation of heat).

The increased leakiness of the blood vessel allows white blood cells, water, and proteins to flow into the area, causing swelling. Often, swelling causes pressure to be exerted on local nerve endings, causing pain.

While macrophages and neutrophils are well adapted to getting the immune system in gear by secreting cytokines, their real job is to get rid of bacteria. They do this by sticking to the bacteria and "swallowing" them, by a process known as **phagocytosis** (phago = eating, cyt = cell) (Figure 6.3). Opsonized bacteria stick to complement receptors, which are proteins on the surface of the macrophage or neutrophil that recognize complement. This causes the **phagocyte** (*i.e.*, macrophage or neutrophil) to engulf the bacterium (Figure 6.4). It does this by encircling the bacterium and enclosing it in a bubble called a **phagosome**. The bacterium is then degraded by a series of potent digestive enzymes and other chemicals that are enclosed in small **granules** that are distributed through the cell. These granules fuse to the phagosome and dump their contents into it with the bacterium, causing the germ to be degraded in a manner not unlike the way food is degraded in the stomach.

Macrophages also use bits of the degraded bacteria to activate the other cells of the immune system, called lymphocytes. Lymphocytes, such as **T cells** and **B cells**, make up what is called the **adaptive immune system** (Figure 6.5); its response is adapted specifically to the organism that is being eliminated. Unlike phagocytes, T cells and B cells do not respond immediately to an invasion. They develop in response to specific activities of the innate immune system.

In order for adaptive immunity to develop, therefore, it must be "informed" by the innate immune system. This occurs when a macrophage, bearing bits of its degraded bacterial meal on its surface, interacts with a certain type of T cell. The degraded bits of bacteria are known as **antigens**, which are recognized by lymphocytes. When the macrophage interacts with

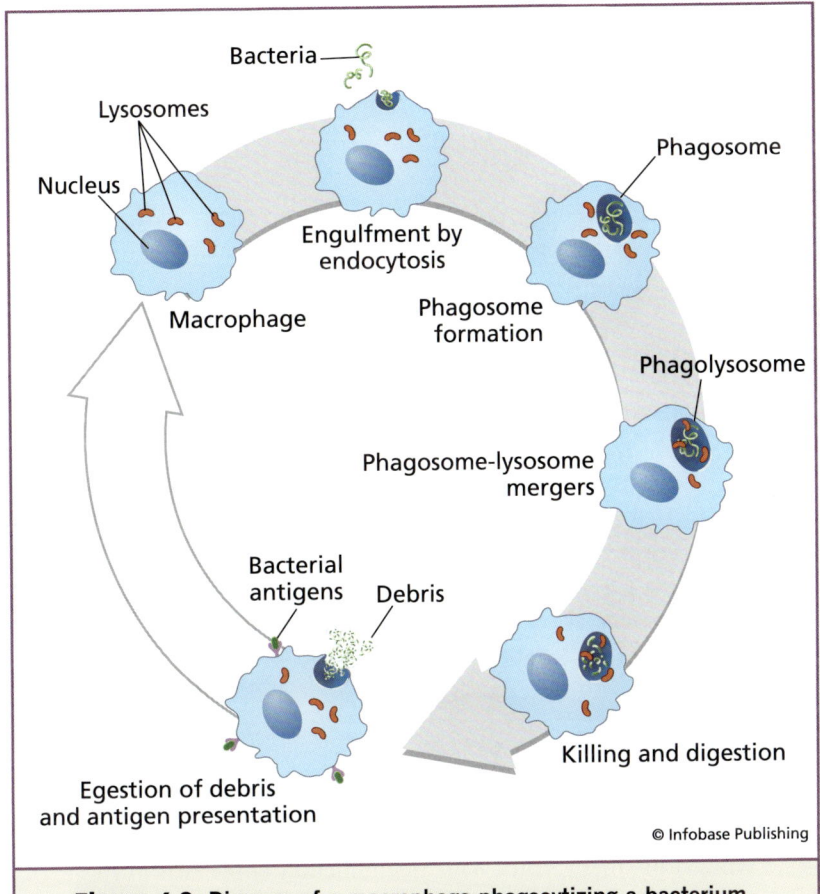

**Figure 6.3** Diagram of a macrophage phagocytizing a bacterium.

a T cell that recognizes the antigen on the macrophage's surface, it will become activated.

Activated T cells then activate B cells that also recognize the same antigen, leading to the production of **antibodies**, which are specific proteins that recognize the antigen presented by the T cell, and only that specific antigen. This aspect of the immune system is highly specific to a particular antigen, and is thus not instantaneously initiated; production of antibodies takes time (up to a few weeks).

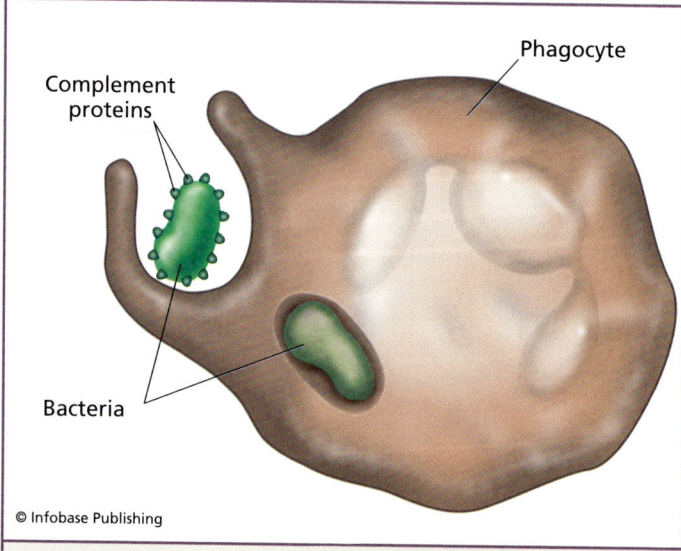

Complement
proteins

Phagocyte

Bacteria

© Infobase Publishing

**Figure 6.4** Diagram illustrating how a phagocyte engulfs a bacterium. Opsonized bacteria bearing complement bound to their outer walls are engulfed by the phagocyte and eliminated.

Once made, activated B cells have a long residence in the body, and continue to make antibodies to combat the specific antigen for many years. This phenomenon is the reason that vaccines are so effective at preventing certain (but not all) illnesses. The B cells, once stimulated by antigens from a particular organism, hang around in tissues and await their next exposure to the antigen. The next time they "see" the antigen, they can rapidly begin to churn out antibodies, helping eliminate the organism and prevent the infection from becoming established.

It is this "memory" function of B cells that vaccines exploit in the prevention of disease. Antibodies produced by B cells in response to a vaccine live in the body for many years, and continue to respond each time the person's body "sees" the organism again.

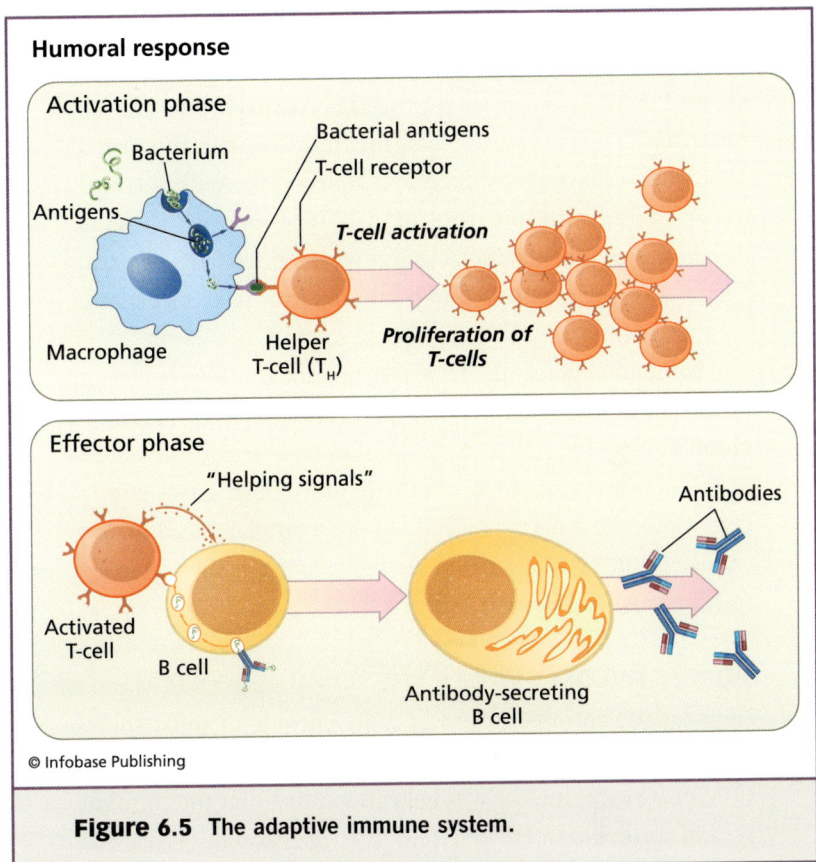

**Humoral response**

**Activation phase**

Bacterial antigens

Bacterium

T-cell receptor

Antigens

**T-cell activation**

Macrophage

Helper
T-cell (T$_H$)

*Proliferation of
T-cells*

**Effector phase**

"Helping signals"

Antibodies

Activated
T-cell

B cell

Antibody-secreting
B cell

© Infobase Publishing

**Figure 6.5** The adaptive immune system.

## INFLAMMATION ALSO KILLS NORMAL CELLS

Inflammatory cells kill bacteria in a variety of ways, some physical and some chemical. Although essential to the immune response, macrophages and neutrophils can also be harmful in that they fight infections in part by releasing toxic compounds used to kill the invading microorganisms. Among the chemicals responsible for killing and degrading invading bacteria are protein-degrading enzymes, enzymes that degrade DNA, as well as molecules such as **hydrogen peroxide** (the liquid that foams when you apply it to cuts) and nitric oxide, which are highly toxic to cells. In addition to acting inside of the phagocyte, many of the molecules that kill and degrade bacterial cells are also released into the surrounding tissues, causing considerable damage to normal cells. New cells replace dead and dying cells, with a consequent increase in the rate of cell turnover. Thus, while inflammation is beneficial because it eliminates invading bacteria, it is also harmful to the tissue in which the bacteria are growing.

Some infections, like *H. pylori*, are not completely cleared by the immune system. With them, inflammation becomes **chronic**, meaning it lasts for a long time. The chronic nature of this disease leads to some of its more destructive effects. Over time, these destructive changes accumulate, leading to a change in the architecture of the tissue and a reduction in the thickness of the stomach lining.

## HOW *H. PYLORI* EVADES THE IMMUNE SYSTEM

In order for an infection to become chronic, it must somehow escape the immune response by either avoiding detection, or by escaping the arsenal of weapons that the immune system throws at it. During its centuries of cohabitation with humans, *H. pylori* has developed a few unique and very clever defenses against the immune system.

### Avoiding the Weapons

*H. pylori* produces several proteins that are toxic to the cells of the stomach lining, and those manufacturing activities alert the immune system to the presence of the invading organism. As described in Chapter 5, proteins such as CagA, which breaks down the junctions between adjacent cells, and VacA, which causes large bubble-like vacuoles to form in the epithelial cells, lead to disruption of the tissue and cell death. As the infection proceeds, sick cells signal to the immune system via a cytokine called Interleukin-8 (IL-8). This cytokine draws in immune cells from the surrounding areas and initiates a large-scale immune invasion.

Macrophages arrive in response to calls from dead and dying cells and begin their attack. However, their efforts are not entirely effective. Under normal circumstances one of the most effective weapons they have against bacteria is the antibacterial agent, nitric oxide (NO). The amino acid L-arginine is required to make this substance. *H. pylori*, however, produces an enzyme called **arginase**, which depletes the L-arginine from the tissue, thereby preventing macrophages from launching their antibacterial chemical assault.

Other bacterial proteins also help *H. pylori* to escape the immune system. In addition to its role in obtaining nutrients from the epithelial cells, the VacA protein produced by *H. pylori* impairs the immune response by making T cells less capable of responding to cytokine signaling. VacA blocks activities of T cell cytokines that tell the T cells to proliferate, and also impairs their interaction with B cells (thereby impairing production of anti-*H. pylori* antibodies).

## Hiding in the Enemy's Camp: *H. pylori* as a Cellular Parasite

In addition to directly blocking the activities of the immune system in hand-to-hand combat, *H. pylori* has found ways to escape notice by the immune system. The immune system is slow to react to bacteria that live inside the host's own cells, so if the invading organism can find its way into these cells, it has time to become well established before being detected and attacked. *H. pylori* has a couple of niches in which it escapes death by immune cells.

One particularly interesting escape mechanism is its ability to survive inside immune cells themselves. Normally, when bacteria are engulfed by macrophages, they are promptly killed; however, some strains of *H. pylori* apparently produce a protein that inhibits the ability of the immune cell to kill them.

As a result, live bacteria are present inside the immune cell for up to 24 hours. *H. pylori* defends itself by causing the vacuoles in which it is engulfed by the macrophage to fuse together, generating one large vacuole inside of the macrophage that contains many bacteria. These large vacuoles are less efficient at killing bacteria than are numerous small vacuoles. In this way, the bacteria are able to delay being killed. It is unclear whether these bacteria later escape back into the tissue, but the fact that they can survive for several hours suggests that this is a potential reservoir of re-infection.

Another hiding place for *H. pylori* is in the epithelium. *H. pylori* lives within and beneath the mucus layer of the stomach, and a fraction of these organisms (around 10 percent) actually attach to the epithelial cells. This close association often leads to the bacteria being taken into and between epithelial cells. Through the activities of CagA, which breaks down the barriers between epithelial cells, bacteria are provided with crevices between adjacent cells into which they can swim and temporarily hide. Also, through the activities of VacA, a few organisms can be drawn into the epithelial cell itself, from which they can later emerge to re-populate the tissue.

This is beneficial for the bacterium in several respects. Because the immune system is extremely well trained to avoid killing host cells, *H. pylori* can avoid attack by hiding inside them. In addition, antibiotics and other harmful substances that might be present in the stomach are not as effective at reaching the bacteria when the organisms are enclosed within the epithelial cells. Furthermore, internalized bacteria avoid being washed away when the stomach empties its contents into the duodenum. In spite of the advantages of life inside the epithelium, however, the majority (90 percent or more) of *H. pylori* organisms in an infected animal or human appear to be free-living in the stomach, rather than epithelial cell parasites.

## Camouflage

*H. pylori* can also hide from the immune system by expressing certain cell surface proteins, called Lewis Blood Group antigens or **Lewis b antigens**. These proteins are expressed widely throughout the body on a large variety of host cells. *H. pylori* expresses them to trick the immune cells into thinking that the bacteria cells belong to the host. Because the immune system is very careful about turning its weapons upon itself, it is prevented from initiating attacks against the disguised bacteria.

This camouflaging process is a controversial topic, however, as immune reactions do occur as a result of other activities that the bacteria perform, and because other notions about the function of this protein have been suggested. Since the receptor for Lewis antigens is also expressed on the surface of the stomach's epithelial cells, it has been suggested that the real function of this protein is to serve as an anchoring point for the bacterium.

Only a minority of the germs (around 10 percent) actually attach to the epithelium, while the remaining 90 percent are distributed throughout the mucus layer. Thus, it has been argued by some scientists that the Lewis Blood Group proteins are more useful in allowing the bacteria to avoid attack by the immune system than in helping them adhere to the epithelium. Additional work on this subject will undoubtedly reveal more about the function of these proteins in the life cycle of the organism.

# 7

# The Role of *H. pylori* in Cancer and Autoimmune Diseases

**Sylvia is a 42-year-old mother of three. She moved to London from Slovenia** when she was 12 and has been a nurse in a hospital for the last eight years. She has had pain in her stomach for as long as she can remember, but the pain became much worse shortly after her first child was born. She knew that she might be infected with *H. pylori*, but didn't want to undergo testing, and instead attributed the pain to her pregnancy and the stress of being a new mother. Over the ensuing years, she had good days and bad, but in the last year, the good days had come less and less often, so she decided to get tested.

When the blood tests revealed that she had antibodies against *H. pylori* and was anemic, the doctor suggested that she undergo an endoscopic exam. Being a nurse, Sylvia knew what to expect, and though she didn't like the idea, she made the appointment and went for the test. While looking inside her stomach, the doctor found some suspicious tissue, which he removed for biopsy. Upon examining this tissue, the doctor concluded that she had a type of cancer called **MALT lymphoma**, a disease that is associated with *H. pylori* infection.

The diagnosis frightened Sylvia a great deal, but she knew that there was treatment available for this disease. After a complete course of antibiotic treatment and another round of endoscopy and biopsy, her lymphoma had almost gone away. Her doctor has since told her that with additional treatment, it is likely that the lymphoma will be cured. She is still nervous, but she also feels very lucky. Not all of her patients have been that fortunate, and she is thankful that her doctor persuaded her to go for testing before the disease had progressed further.

## *H. PYLORI* AND CANCER

In 1994 the International Agency for Research on Cancer (IARC) declared *H. pylori* a definite carcinogen. This was a big step. Very few "definite" carcinogens have been identified, even though trillions of research dollars have been spent and millions of scientists and physicians have devoted their entire careers to the study and treatment of this disease. This label places *H. pylori* in a class with such infamous agents as cigarette smoke, asbestos, and UV and ionizing radiation. Unfortunately, however, the fact that the label has been applied does not mean that we truly understand how *H. pylori* works its mischief in the production of cancer. What it does mean, though, is that the association between infection and cancer is sufficiently strong (through clinical and epidemiological studies) and the scientific rationale so clear that a definite link can be made.

Before we can begin to understand the role that *H. pylori* may play in causing gastric and duodenal cancer and intestinal lymphoma, we must first discuss what cancer is and how it forms. Although we tend to discuss cancer as though it were a single disease, cancer is not really *one* disease, it is actually hundreds of diseases, all with different compositions and life histories. In fact, even for a given organ there are different types of cancer that may form, depending on the cells involved and the process that the tissue underwent during development of the disease. An example of this is skin cancer, which can include melanoma (a disease of the pigment-producing cells of the skin) and basal cell carcinoma (a disease of the skin's basal cells). What makes this more complicated is that, even for a

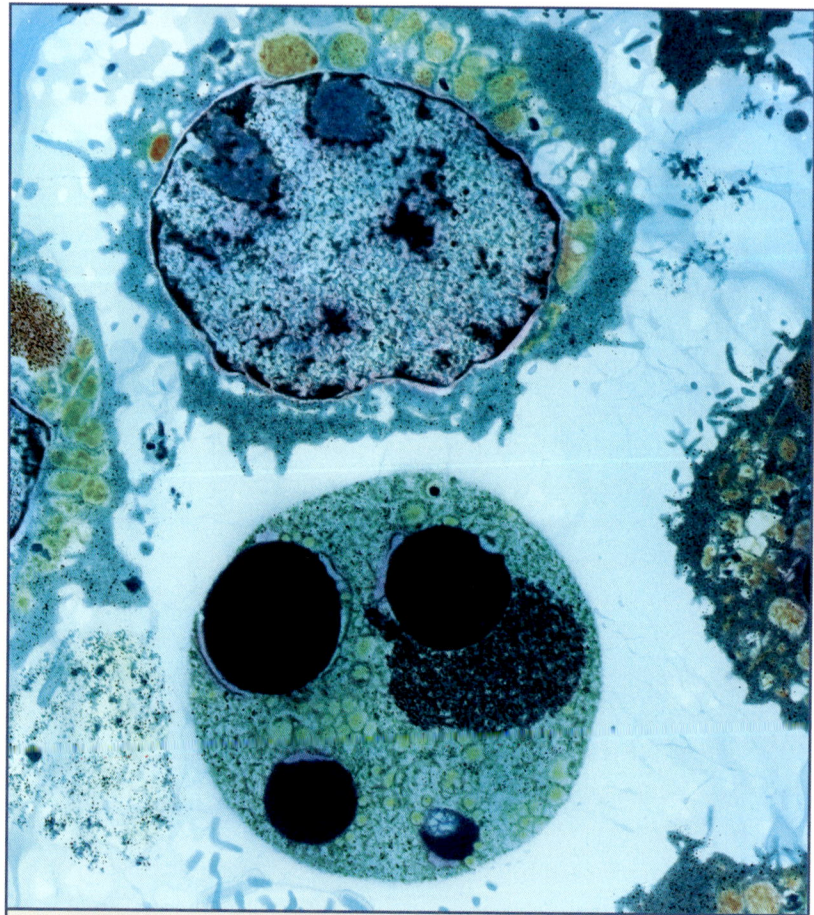

**Figure 7.1** Colored transmission electron micrograph (TEM) of a healthy white blood cell (lower center) during apoptosis. (Dr. Gobal Murti/Photo Researchers, Inc.)

given type of cancer, each case is as unique as the person who harbors it.

So, what is cancer? Cancer is a disease in which the cells of an organ or tissue lose their ability to recognize the normal signals that the body and neighboring cells send out to direct their growth, function, and death. Under normal circumstances, a balance of cell growth and cell death keeps the size of the cell population more or less constant. This cell death is a key physiological process known as **apoptosis** (Figure 7.1). An appropriate balance of cell growth and apoptosis is a crucial dynamic in the maintenance of healthy tissue, and cancerous tissues typically have alterations in one or both of these processes, that is, increased cell growth and/or decreased apoptosis.

The structure of the tissue is also crucial in keeping its cells functioning properly. Normal cells in healthy tissue maintain tight physical connections to their neighbors and respond to signals that they receive from the blood or adjacent cells. And, except for those in a few tissues (e.g., hair, intestine, blood), constituent cells do not divide rapidly;  they divide only in response to the death or injury of a neighboring cell. This close physical and chemical communication instructs cells regarding what the tissue and organism require, and closely regulates their behavior.

In contrast, cancer cells often lose their physical connection to adjacent cells and thereby lose their physical communication, and their ability to receive chemical signals from the blood and body fluids. As a result, the cancer cells become isolated and often begin to proliferate and function differently from the other tissues in the organ. These cancerous cells can do a variety of bizarre things. They may begin to look differently or take on the function of a different cell type (for example, an abnormal stomach cell may begin to look and function like a pancreatic or intestinal cell—a process known as **metaplasia**, an adaptive change that can be but is not always pre-cancerous), or they may migrate into the circulatory or lymphatic systems and travel to another organ, creating new colonies elsewhere (a process called **metastasis**).

All of this cellular anarchy leads to a loss of normal function in the tissue. Thus, the normal cells of the tissue, most of which do not divide rapidly, are pushed aside or are otherwise squeezed out and replaced by cells that function abnormally, divide too rapidly, and are resistant to apoptosis. The organ then loses its function and the person who carries the tumor begins to exhibit symptoms of its failure.

Cancer is usually defined by its location (brain cancer, liver cancer, breast cancer, etc.), by the microscopic appearance of its cells, and by the degree to which it has spread (or metastasized). This geographic type of division makes sense; knowing in which organ the cancer has developed tells the physician a good deal about the disease's life history and likely outcome. It also reveals something about how it could have arisen. For example, lung cancer in a smoker is not surprising, nor is melanoma in a sun-worshipper.

## GENES AND CANCER

The underlying cause of any cancer is a change in the normal pattern of gene expression. The genes that are expressed by each cell type in the body define that cell type, in that genes direct the pattern of protein expression. Proteins are a major type of structural and functional molecule in the body, and make up more than 15 percent of the cell's total content. They compose the skeleton of the cell, a large portion of the outer membrane, almost all of the enzymes that direct the cell's chemical reactions, energy production, growth and proliferation, and many of the substances that are secreted into the blood stream to support the body's normal physiology (such as insulin).

Most cancer biologists believe that the changes in gene expression that lead to cancer occur in multiple stages, a theory called the **multistage model of carcinogenesis** (Figure 7.2). This theory proposes that several things must happen to make a normal cell transform into a cancerous cell. First, it must acquire gene mutations that inactivate growth-suppressing genes (so-called **tumor suppressors**) and/or activate growth-promoting genes (so-called **oncogenes**). This stage is called **initiation**, and appears to involve a change to the cell's DNA.

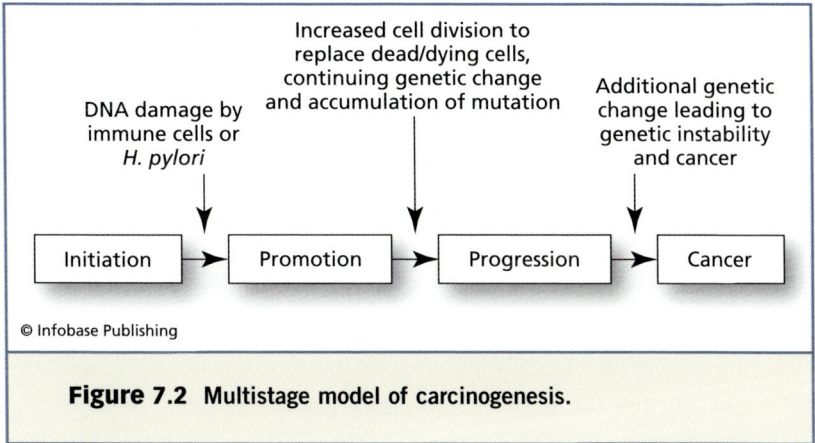

**Figure 7.2** Multistage model of carcinogenesis.

Agents that induce mutations in genes are called **mutagens**. These agents differ widely in their makeup and activity. They may be chemicals (like benzene), viruses (like human papilloma virus or hepatitis C), bacteria (like *H. pylori*), other agents like asbestos (a mineral fiber once used in insulation), or ionizing or UV radiation. Different classes of mutagens may act very differently in the precise manner by which they cause mutations. Some act directly on DNA, such as benzene, which damages DNA, or radiation, which breaks DNA; others, like *H. pylori*, act both directly and indirectly, as we shall see shortly.

The next step in the process of carcinogenesis is called **promotion**. This can be a non-mutational change that sets the cellular replication machinery in motion by triggering chemical reactions inside the cell that tell it to replicate its DNA and divide. By itself, excess replication does not lead to cancer; it is just one way by which most mutated cells expand their numbers. However, it is the genetic events that occur during and after that expansion of mutated cells that actually lead to the development of cancer.

As the cells are prompted to divide, the genetic changes may continue to occur and accumulate. The cell's genetic material thus becomes less intact and increasingly "unstable," leading to greater and greater genetic disorganization. During this process, the cell makes the transition from healthy to malignant, a process known as **progression**.

## H. PYLORI AND GASTRIC CANCER

Gastric (stomach) cancer is the second most common type of cancer in the world. Most cancers of the stomach arise in the antrum, which is the lower third of the stomach, near the duodenum. There are different kinds of stomach cancers, depending on the type of cells from which the cancer arises. Cancers that form in the stomach's secretory glands are called **adenocarcinomas**; these are the most common form, accounting for more than 90 percent of all stomach cancers. Other types are **sarcomas** (cancers of the stomach's muscle layer), and **gastric lymphomas**, which form in certain immune cells (B and T cells) of the stomach tissue.

Adenocarcinoma of the stomach is strongly associated with *H. pylori* infection. Recent studies of patients with stomach cancer have revealed that over 90 percent of people who develop adenocarcinoma of the stomach have *H. pylori* infections. So, what is it about *H. pylori* that predisposes certain people to develop cancer? A recent theory on the development of stomach cancer revolves around the interaction between the *H. pylori* organism itself and the infected person's own immune response.

## H. PYLORI GENES, HOST IMMUNITY, AND THE FORMATION OF ADENOCARCINOMA

The role of *H. pylori* in the development of stomach cancer fits the multi-stage theory of carcinogenesis very well. There are two important factors in the formation of gastric cancer, and it is likely that they act in a cooperative manner to produce the cancerous changes.

First, the host's own immune system, which releases bacteria-killing products as it battles infection, causes damage to the DNA of the stomach lining's cells (initiation). Second, the bacterium itself and the products that it makes may directly injure or kill the cells lining the stomach, leading to an increased turnover rate of cells in the tissue (promotion), a decreased rate of cell death (apoptosis), and a change in gene expression that leads to a shift away from normal stomach cell functioning.

The strain of *H. pylori* to which a person is exposed may influence the risk of developing gastric cancer. Strains of *H. pylori* that produce high levels of two proteins, vacuolating toxin A (VacA) and the cytotoxin-associated gene A (CagA), appear to cause greater tissue damage than those that produce lower levels, or that lack those genes completely. These proteins are directly toxic to cells lining the stomach, and signal strongly to the immune system that an invasion is underway. As a result of the bacterial presence, neutrophils and macrophages set up residence in the tissue to fight the bacteria assault.

Macrophages and neutrophils produce a number of substances that are destructive to neighboring cells, and that may in fact lead to mutations in the DNA of tissue cells. One of these substances is nitric oxide (NO), an antibacterial product that is made by neutrophils and dumped into the surrounding area to cleanse the region of invading microbes. NO, however, is a powerful oxidizing agent (similar to hydrogen peroxide); the activity of these strong oxidants causes small breaks in the DNA of the cells immediately surrounding the neutrophil.

These breaks can lead to a loss of genes (such as tumor suppressors), a rearrangement of genes, or to other genetic mutations that change how the protein functions (including, for example, permanent activation of oncogenes, which promote cell growth, or inactivation of genes that stop cell growth). Indeed, a number of gastric cancers have been observed to cause a loss of the tumor suppressor function, an activation of oncogenes, and changes in many other genes that regulate the rate of cell growth and apoptosis.

These changes in DNA and gene expression are also reflected in the re-organization of cells in the tissues—

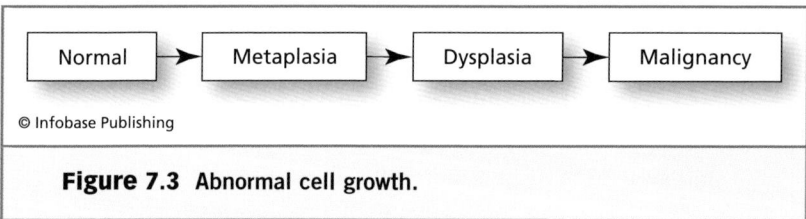

© Infobase Publishing

**Figure 7.3** Abnormal cell growth.

a re-organization that can be seen through a microscope. The destruction of cells in the stomach tissue results in a condition known as **gastric atrophy**. Gastric atrophy can then progress to another state known as **intestinal metaplasia,** in which epithelial cells lining the stomach take on different characteristics, and thus the organization of the tissue becomes more like that of the intestine than the stomach. The stomach tissue's loss of function that stems from this re-organization is believed to be an early indicator that all is not well in that region. The risk of gastric cancer increases rapidly as the degree of inflammation and metaplasia increases.

As metaplasia worsens, the tissue takes on a more disorganized appearance and function. So now, instead of behaving like intestinal cells, the cells become more disordered and eventually reach a state called **dysplasia,** a more dangerous condition in which the cells ignore most of the rules that govern cell growth and function (Figure 7.3). The result is a chaotic state of excess growth, invasion, and spread. This is thought to be the last step before the tissue becomes truly cancerous. The transition from metaplasia to cancer may involve additional genetic rearrangements, including loss of more tumor suppressors and activation of more oncogenes.

Eventually, the dysplastic tissue may become cancerous, or **malignant**. Malignant cells may then gain the ability to move out of their immediate vicinity to more distant sites. They do this by entering the circulatory or lymph systems, by which they are carried to other organs, such as the liver or pancreas. This process is known as **metastasis**. There, the cells form metastatic colonies that hijack the function of the organ to which they have spread. So, for example, if the gastric adenocarcinoma metastasizes to the liver, cancer cells replace normal liver cells in the region of the liver where the cancer is growing. That area then ceases to function like liver tissue, and begins to function like the cancer tissue that has replaced it.

This is a very serious stage in the life cycle of the disease, a stage at which medical treatment becomes more difficult. As with most cancers, early intervention improves the outcome. Early diagnosis and medical treatment are very important in helping a person to recover from gastric cancer.

## *H. PYLORI* AND MALT LYMPHOMA

In addition to gastric adenocarcinoma, there are other cancers associated with *H. pylori* infection. The most important of these is **MALT lymphoma**, which is a tumor of the mucosa-associated lymphoid tissue. MALT is essentially an accumulation of immune cells that are distributed throughout the stomach epithelium in long-standing *H. pylori* infections.

The formation of *H. pylori*-associated MALT lymphoma is believed to occur in a fashion similar to that of gastric adenocarcinoma. Like adenocarcinoma formation, the bacterial presence results in long-standing tissue inflammation. This inflammation leads to changes in resident lymphocytes (T or B cells, primarily) and shifts the balance of cell division and apoptosis such that the lymphocytes begin to accumulate at an abnormally high level in certain spots. These high concentrations of lymphocytes displace normal cells, leading to areas of abnormal tissue with reduced function. Increased expression of oncogenes, which promote cell growth, and reduced apoptosis have been documented in samples taken from patients with this condition.

## AUTOIMMUNITY

Besides cancer and stomach ulcers, *H. pylori* infection has also been tied to various autoimmune diseases. **Autoimmune**

**diseases** are those in which the immune system begins to attack normal cells in the body. Although many autoimmune diseases have been linked to *H. pylori* infection, most of the theories on this subject are very controversial.

## *HELICOBACTER PYLORI* AND THE FORMATION OF AUTO-ANTIBODIES

*H. pylori* infection can lead to the production of **auto-antibodies**, which are antibodies directed against the infected person's own cells. This can occur if the antibody produced in response to the *H. pylori* organism also recognizes, or **cross-reacts** with, the normal cells of the body.

One well-established link between *H. pylori* and auto-antibody formation occurs in the production of antibodies against proteins in the cells of the stomach. These antibodies can bind to the stomach's cells and elicit a destructive immune response by inflammatory cells in the stomach tissue, leading to elimination of the antibody-bound cell. This is believed to be one way by which *H. pylori* infection leads to the onset of gastric atrophy. If antibodies recognize cells of the gastric mucosa, they will cause immune destruction of the cells lining the stomach. In one study conducted in Japan, more than half of the *H. pylori*-infected patients that were studied had antibodies in their blood that recognized normal stomach cells.

A hypothesis that is less well-established is the link between *H. pylori* and autoimmune thyroid disease. Studies of people with autoimmune thyroid disease have hinted that, in some people, antibodies may cross-react with cells of the thyroid gland, causing destruction of thyroid tissue. Because the thyroid gland secretes thyroid hormones that help regulate the rate of metabolism, destruction of the thyroid gland may lead to a reduction in thyroid hormones and thus a slower metabolic rate.

*H. pylori* has also been linked to various blood disorders. One study suggests that *H. pylori* is associated with the formation of antibodies against the body's own neutrophils. This condition is thought to cause reduced levels of neutrophils in the blood, a condition known as **autoimmune neutropenia.** In this study, elimination of *H. pylori* reduced the amount of auto-antibodies in the blood and restored the normal number of neutrophils. However, this is still a controversial theory.

A reduction in blood platelets, the cells in the blood that are responsible for blood clotting, has also been tied to *H. pylori* and the formation of auto-antibodies. Antibodies that react against platelets cause them to be destroyed by the immune system, thereby lowering their number in the blood, a condition known as **immune thrombocytopenia purpura (ITP).** This is a very dangerous condition that can lead to excessive bruising and bleeding, and can also cause a person to bleed to death if they sustain a serious injury or cut. ITP is considered a medical emergency, but treatments are available to suppress the immune reaction that causes the disease. Despite the severity of this disease, it is not known what causes the immune system to form antibodies against its platelets. While *H. pylori*-associated auto-antibodies have been suggested as one possible cause, this link is still debated, and additional studies are underway to test this idea.

# 8

# Diagnosis and Treatment of *H. pylori*

Andrei is a 16-year-old high school sophomore who has been suffering from a sore, upset stomach for over a year. He and his parents emigrated from Russia when he was six years old, and both parents have undergone ulcer treatment in the past few years. Andrei has always had a healthy appetite, but lately the pain in his stomach that occurs just after he eats has made him avoid eating. He has lost weight, is frequently tired, and has a hard time concentrating at school. His food intake has diminished to less than half of its previous level because he simply isn't hungry most of the time. He tries to avoid spicy and high-protein foods, which seem to make the pain worse, but even that isn't working any more.

The doctor listened to him carefully and asked many questions about where the pain is located, what it feels like, and when it happens. He also wanted to know about Andrei's family history of stomach pain and about any other family members who have had ulcers or stomach cancer. When Andrei had finished, the doctor told him that he might be infected with *H. pylori*; he explained that the infection is common in Russia and that Andrei probably became infected as a child. The doctor continued by asking Andrei to undergo an endoscopic examination of his stomach, and promising that, if *H. pylori* was the cause of his stomach pain, he could very likely be cured with a simple course of antibiotic treatment.

The chief complaint among people infected with *H. pylori* is **dyspepsia** (also called indigestion), which is a condition characterized by upper abdominal pain (above the navel), nausea, vomiting, bloating, and

96

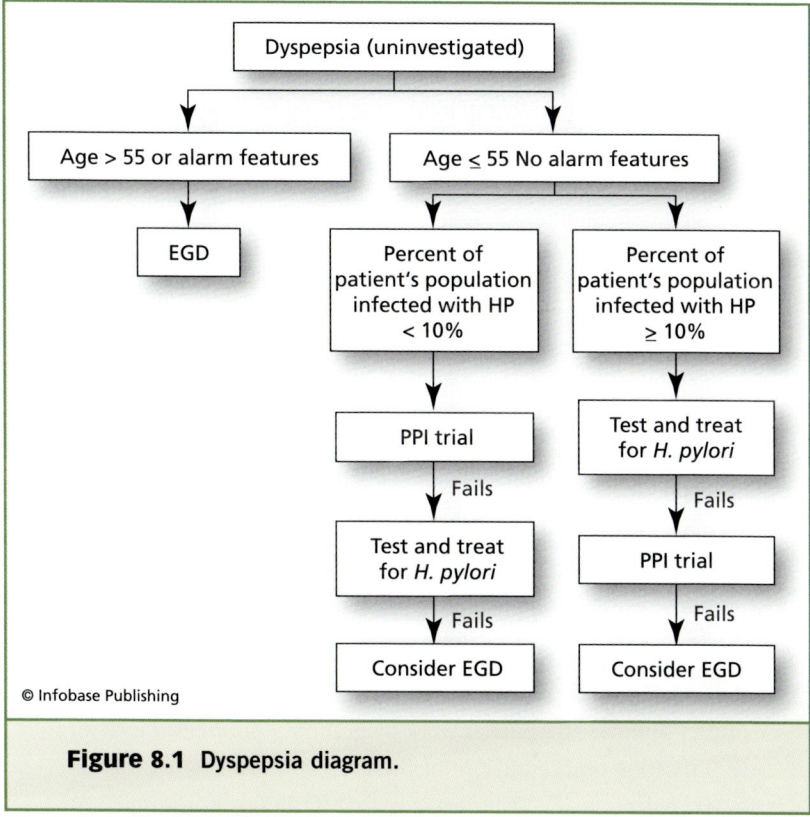

**Figure 8.1** Dyspepsia diagram.

abdominal swelling, and may be accompanied by a sense of excessive fullness even after eating small amounts of food. The symptoms of dyspepsia are most often triggered by meals, and certain types of food may worsen the condition. If the infection progresses to a more serious condition, the dyspeptic symptoms may also be accompanied by an intense gnawing or burning pain in the stomach, as well as tiredness and anemia, symptoms that may indicate that an ulcer has formed. (Figure 8.1)

When a patient complains to his or her physician about dyspepsia and stomach pain, the doctor may want to investigate further to rule out other conditions or lifestyle factors that may be causing the symptoms. The first question may be whether the patient is a heavy user of aspirin or NSAIDs, which may by themselves cause ulcers. If the answer is "no," the doctor may ask other questions about the patient's diet, lifestyle, ethnic background, and family history.

## HOW PROTON PUMP INHIBITORS WORK

Gastric fluid contains a high concentration of hydrochloric acid (HCl). When in an aqueous (water-based) solution, HCl separates into two electrically charged atoms called ions, resulting in the production of a positively charged hydrogen ion ($H^+$) and a negatively charged chloride ion ($Cl^-$). Hydrogen ions ($H^+$), also called protons, make the gastric fluid acidic. Acids are solutions that contain an abundance of protons.

$$HCl \longrightarrow H^+ + Cl^-$$

The parietal cells secrete this acid into the stomach with the aid of specialized, membrane-embedded proteins called proton pumps. The pumps work by grabbing potassium ions ($K^+$) that are on the outside of the cell, and exchanging them for $H^+$ on the inside. The result is that $K^+$ is taken into the cell, and $H^+$ is pushed out of the cell and into the lumen of the stomach. The action of these pumps is turned on in response to a meal, and used to activate the digestive enzymes of the stomach.

Proton pump inhibitors (PPIs), such as omeprazole (Prilosec), work by inhibiting the activity of those pumps, and thereby reduce the acidity of the stomach environment. However, because not all of the pumps are structurally identical, the PPI does not inhibit all of them, and there is still sufficient acidity to allow digestion to occur. The reduced acidity, however, does allow ulcerated regions in the stomach to heal, and preserves the activity of antibiotics that may be needed to treat an *H. pylori* infection.

If the overall frequency of *H. pylori* in the population is low (as it is in most developed countries), it may not be the first thing that the physician considers unless the patient has a known risk factor for infection. Known risk factors include emigration from a country with a high prevalence of infection, having infected household members, or belonging to an ethnic group that is known to have a higher-than-average infection rate. If any of those risk factors apply, the doctor may opt to test the patient for *H. pylori*. If not, the doctor may decide to treat the dyspepsia symptoms without testing the patient for infection.

Specialized drugs called **proton pump** inhibitors (PPIs) such as Prilosec (omeprazole) and Nexium (esomeprazole), which inhibit the acid production mechanism in the stomach, have been developed to treat dyspepsia and are often quite effective for relieving symptoms in people who do not have an *H. pylori* infection. In patients for whom there is no known risk factor for *H. pylori* infection, this may be the first treatment for dyspepsia. In patients for whom PPIs do not alleviate symptoms, and in those with known risk factors for *H. pylori* infection, the doctor may order tests to determine whether the patient is infected with *H. pylori* and to evaluate the extent of the damage.

### DIAGNOSING AN *H. PYLORI* INFECTION

There are a number of tests available to diagnose *H. pylori* infections. The tests differ in their accuracy and sensitivity, and not all are equally suitable for everyone. There are two basic classes of tests: invasive and non-invasive.

An invasive test is usually reserved for young children and patients whose symptoms suggest a cause for serious concern. In an adult, symptoms that suggest a severe ulcer with complications might warrant a more invasive examination. These alarm symptoms include: advanced age, a long history of symptoms, persistent weight loss or lack of appetite, gastrointestinal bleeding (tarry, black stools), anemia, persistent vomiting, and severe stomach pain. This type of test not only diagnoses the amount of damage in the stomach, but also allows the physician to directly sample the tissue to test it for the presence of the *H. pylori* organism.

Non-invasive tests are those that can detect the presence of the *H. pylori* organism, but do not reveal as much about the tissue damage that the organism may have caused. Non-invasive tests use other, less direct means to determine whether the organism is present, such as testing for the presence of antibodies to *H. pylori* or the presence of *H. pylori* urease. These biochemical tests may be less reliable than endoscopy in diagnosing the infection, as they sometimes fail to detect the organism in an infected person (false negative) or incorrectly diagnose an uninfected person (false positive).

## INVASIVE TESTS
### Histological Examination

An invasive test is the most accurate available, and are the most widely accepted for diagnosing *H. pylori* in young children. The invasive test is called esophagogastroduodenoscopy (EGD), so named because it allows the physician to view the esophagus, stomach, and duodenum. The endoscope, which is used for the invasive test, is a flexible tube equipped with a camera and small surgical tools. During the exam, the physician inserts an endoscope down the patient's throat into the stomach. Pictures from the camera are relayed to a video monitor, allowing the physician to directly observe the tissue lining the stomach and duodenum. The endoscopically operated surgical instruments can then be used to collect tissue specimens.

Once the damaged area is identified, a sample can be retrieved and sent to a pathologist for microscopic examination. *H. pylori*-infected tissue usually exhibits symptoms of inflammation (neutrophils and lymphocytes). In long-standing infections, the organism may not be easily seen, so the pathologist may need to use special tissue stains. However, the presence of inflammation is easily observed and is a key diagnostic criterion. If an endoscopic biopsy reveals that the stomach lining is normal and free of inflammatory cells, other types of ulcers, such as those caused by NSAIDS, may be considered more likely.

## Culturing *H. pylori*

Successful culture of the *H. pylori* organism is the gold standard for diagnosis. The bacterium can be recovered from biopsy specimens and grown in the laboratory, though recovering the *H. pylori* bacteria from tissue requires prompt handling of the sample and specialized equipment and training. As a result, this is rarely done except in cases that are difficult to treat. Most pathologists thus rely on other criteria—such as the degree of inflammation of the tissue, or perhaps observing the organism in the tissue—for diagnosis.

## Rapid Urease Test (RUT)

The rapid urease test is used to detect the presence of the *H. pylori* urease enzyme. One of the small pieces of biopsied tissue from the stomach's antrum is placed in a liquid containing urea and a chemical that changes color in response to alterations in the acidity of the solution. If *H. pylori* is present, it will metabolize the urea to produce ammonia. Because ammonia makes the liquid less acidic and the indicator dye is sensitive to changes in acid level, the solution will change color in the presence of *H. pylori*.

There are several versions of this test, and most use some variation of this method to detect the *H. pylori* organism in fresh tissue. This type of test is quite sensitive and specific for *H. pylori*, but versions of the tests vary in terms of how long they take to detect the organism. For some tests, a result can be obtained in as few as 20 minutes, while in others it can take more than 24 hours. In patients without complications, this test can substitute for microscopic examination by a pathologist.

In borderline cases, the other bits of tissue obtained from the endoscopic exam can be sent to the pathologist for microscopic examination. This backup option allows for verification of ambiguous results without subjecting the patient to a second round of endoscopy.

## NON-INVASIVE TESTS
### Blood Tests

As described in previous chapters, infection with *H. pylori* elicits a strong immune response that results in the production of antibodies, which can be detected in the blood. In many cases, a simple blood test will tell a doctor whether a person has had an *H. pylori* infection. A positive antibody test, accompanied by dyspeptic symptoms, may be enough information for the doctor to prescribe antibiotic therapy to eradicate the *H. pylori* infection.

One problem with this blood test, however, is that the presence of *H. pylori*-fighting antibodies does not necessarily indicate that the person has an active infection. Antibodies can remain in the circulation for many months or years after an infection has been eliminated by the immune system. Under these circumstances, a positive blood test can lead to misdiagnosis and improper treatment.

### Urea Breath Test

One of the more clever tests to detect *H. pylori* is the urea breath test (Figure 8.2). This test makes use of the fact that *H. pylori* produces urease, an enzyme that metabolizes urea into ammonia and carbon dioxide ($CO_2$), which is a gas. For this test, patients swallow a capsule that contains a small amount of $^{13}C$-labeled urea. $^{13}C$ is a special form of carbon that is slightly heavier than normal carbon. The $^{13}CO_2$ is absorbed through the stomach lining and transported to the circulatory system where it is exhaled through the lungs and measured by a machine. Patients who do not have *H. pylori* infections will produce little or no $^{13}CO_2$, and the urea will be metabolized by the body and eliminated in the feces and urine. This is not only a good diagnostic test, but also a good means of evaluating whether a course of *H. pylori* therapy has successfully eradicated the organism; however, this test may be less reliable for children.

## Fecal Antigen Test

The fecal antigen test is used to detect *H. pylori* proteins and other antigens in the feces of patients who are suspected of having an active *H. pylori* infection. For this test, small fecal

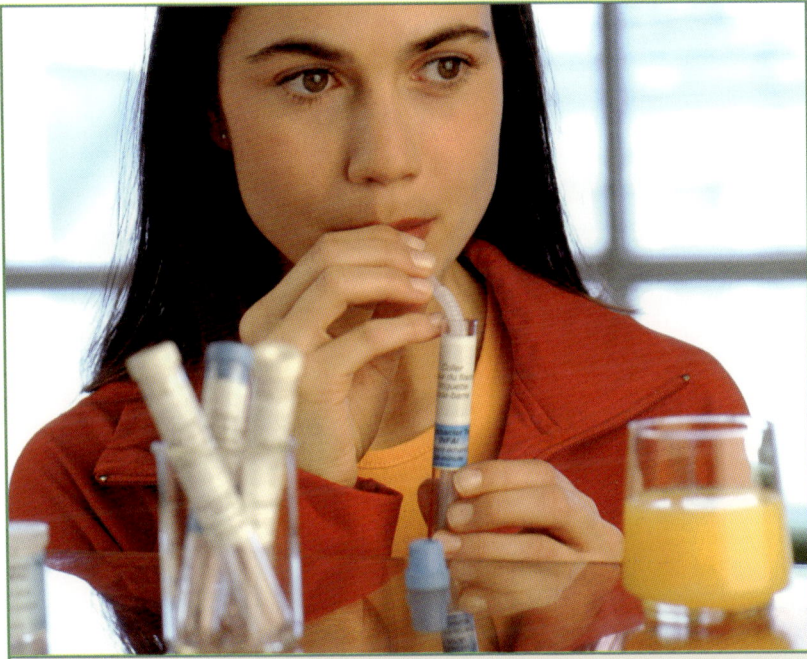

**Figure 8.2** A patient blows into a sample tube during a urea breath test for gastric ulcers caused by bacteria. (GARO/Photo Researchers, Inc.)

samples from the patient are mixed with chemicals that change color in the presence of the antigens. The test is highly sensitive and specific, and is especially good for children.

**Table 8.1** Comparison of Tests for *Helicobacter pylori.*

| Test | Advantages | Disadvantages |
|---|---|---|
| Endoscopy | Very accurate, especially for young children<br>Allows evaluation of damage to stomach and duodenum | Recent use of proton pump inhibitors, bisthmus, or antibiotics affects results<br>Must be performed in a clinic or hospital |
| *H. pylori* culture | Diagnostic | Requires endoscopic examination<br>Expensive, difficult to perform and not widely available<br>Because of technical problems with this method, many infections fail to be diagnosed |
| Urease Test | Sensitive and accurate | Requires endoscopic examination<br>Sensitivity may be lower in patients with GI bleeding |
| Urea Breath Test | Sensitive and accurate<br>Non-invasive | May be less reliable in children |
| *H. pylori* Blood Test | Non invasive | Sensitive<br>Does not distinguish between active and previous infection |
| Stool Antigen Text | Sensitive and accurate<br>Non-invasive<br>Inexpensive | None |

## TREATMENT OF *H. PYLORI* INFECTIONS

So, how does an infected person get rid of an *H. pylori* infection? Once an *H. pylori* infection is diagnosed, it is usually treated with what is called a "triple-combination therapy," which consists of two antibiotics plus a proton pump inhibitor. These are administered twice daily for seven to 14 days. There are a number of antibiotics that are commonly used, including amoxicillin, clarithromycin, metronidazole, and tetracycline, among many others.

The purpose of a triple-combination treatment regimen is two-fold. First, two antibiotics are used to ensure that the bacterium doesn't develop antibiotic resistance during treatment. *H. pylori* becomes antibiotic resistant quite easily through changes in its DNA; however, while it is relatively easy to escape one antibiotic, it is virtually impossible to escape two at the same time. Secondly, because the infection is located in the stomach and most antibiotics are not stable in an acidic environment, a PPI is added, which extends the life of the antibiotics at the site where they are most needed. Provided that the infected person's bacterial strain is not resistant to the antibiotics, this regimen successfully cures, or **eradicates**, over 90 percent of the infections on which it is used.

## WHY DON'T DOCTORS JUST TREAT EVERYONE? CONSEQUENCES OF ANTIBIOTIC RESISTANCE

You may be wondering why doctors don't just treat everyone for *H. pylori* infection. After all, the organism is responsible for a tremendous amount of suffering and death worldwide. Why not just get rid of it? This is an attractive idea, and it has certainly been discussed in the scientific and medical communities; however, it is not currently practical to treat everyone in the world for *H. pylori*.

There are a number of reasons why this is true. First, antibiotic therapy is not without risks. Serious, life-threatening allergic reactions to antibiotics are relatively common, so it would be unethical to expose people to what could be a serious risk without adequate justification (like a diagnosis of infection with *H. pylori*). Secondly, antibiotic resistance is becoming

## ELISA AND THE FECAL ANTIGEN TEST

The fecal antigen test uses a type of technique called an ELISA (enzyme-linked immunosorbent assay). This test makes use of the fact that antibodies made against a particular antigen recognize that and only that one antigen. Antibodies used in this test are made in animals (such as cows, sheep, or rabbits) by injecting the animal with extracts of *H. pylori*. Purified *H. pylori* antibodies are then dried onto the bottom of small wells in a cell culture dish (Figure 8.3, Panel 1). Small fecal samples from a patient suspected of having an active *H. pylori* infection are diluted in liquid and added to the culture dish (Figure 8.3, Panel 2). If the patient is infected with *H. pylori*, antigens present in the feces will bind to the antibodies. After a few minutes, the liquid is removed and the dish is washed to remove excess material that did not bind to the antibodies; the antibodies and their bound material remain in the bottom of the dish. A second antibody, which is attached to an enzyme, is then added to the well and allowed to bind (Figure 8.3, Panel 3). This creates an "antigen sandwich," in which two anti-*H. pylori* antibodies are stuck together by a thin layer of antigen. After a few minutes, the unbound antibody is washed away; however, the antigen sandwich is extremely stable and will stay in the well during the washing steps. In the last step, a chemical is added that reacts with the enzyme that is bound to the second antibody (Figure 8.3, Panel 4). This reaction, which will only occur in the presence of antibody-bound *H. pylori* antigens, will produce a bright color in the solution that can be measured by a special machine that quantifies the amount of color produced.

a huge problem in the fight against *H. pylori.* For example, in Germany and the Netherlands over 20 percent of people with *H. pylori* infections carry strains that are resistant to

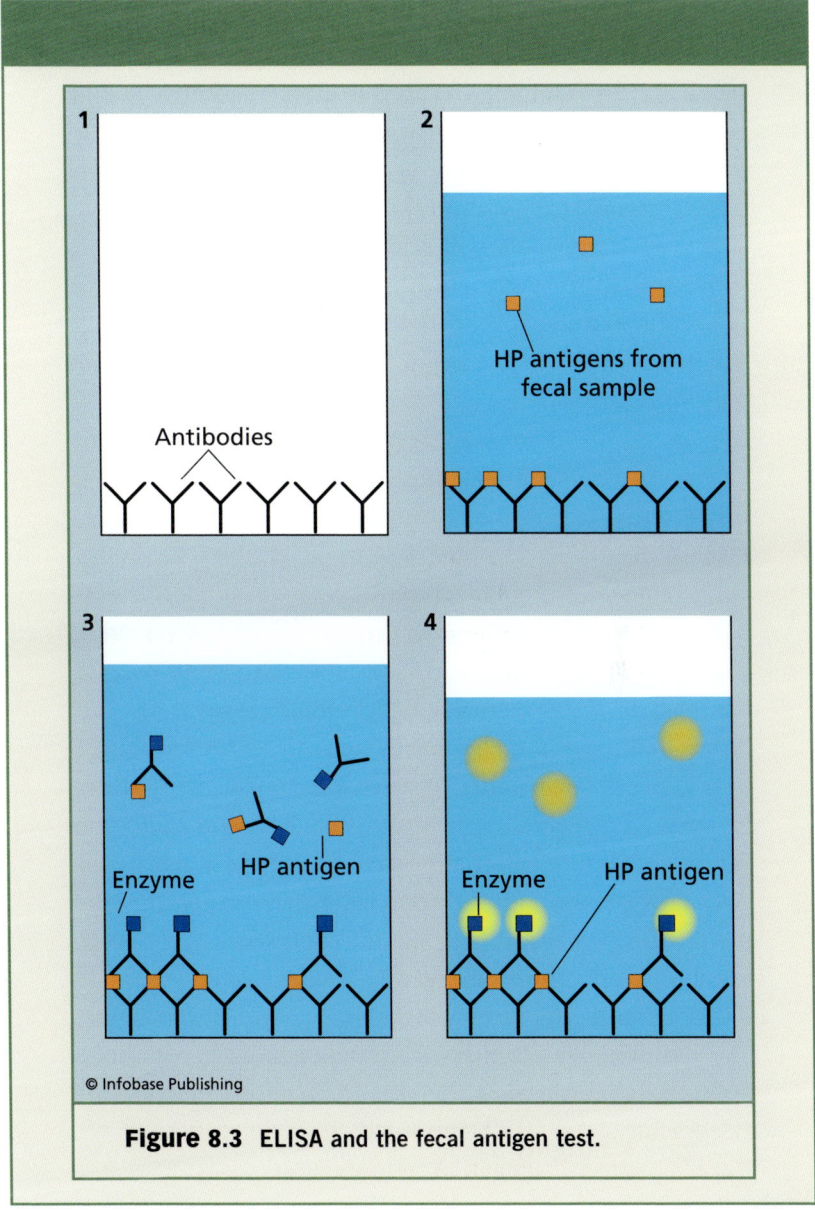

© Infobase Publishing

**Figure 8.3** ELISA and the fecal antigen test.

clarithromycin, one of the most commonly used antibiotics to treat this disease. Similarly, between 20 to 40 percent of strains in Europe and the United States are resistant to metronidazole. This trend is extremely worrisome in terms of the future of *H. pylori* treatment. Efforts are underway to produce new antibiotics and new treatment regimens (triple-antibiotic therapy plus a PPI, for example). The progress is slow, however, and the resulting treatments are more costly and therefore available to fewer people worldwide. For these reasons, effort is made to restrict *H. pylori* eradication therapy to people with demonstrable infection who would benefit most from its use.

## A VACCINE FOR *H. PYLORI*?

Efforts are underway to develop a vaccine for *H. pylori* that not only might prevent new infections, but also might help people who are already infected. So, how would a vaccine help? A vaccine is a mixture of foreign proteins and other molecules that is introduced into the body (usually orally or by injection) to help stimulate the immune system to produce antibodies against those proteins and molecules. So, for example, if a mixture of *H. pylori* proteins were used to vaccinate a person, it would likely cause the body to form antibodies against the proteins that the organism makes, which would cause the immune system of the vaccinated person to attack the germ. This can be used either before or after the person becomes infected with the germ. If it is used before an infection occurs, the infection will be eliminated before it becomes established, and if it is given after a person is already infected, it may further stimulate the immune system to fight the infection more aggressively, possibly curing the infected person. (Figure 8.4)

What are the problems with developing an *H. pylori* vaccine? The best vaccine is one that contains several foreign molecules.

**Figure 8.4 (right)** Vaccine immunity.

**Step 1:**

Antigens specific to the disease-causing organism are injected into the body.

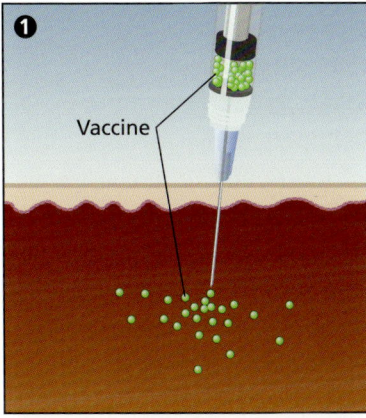

**Step 2:**

Antibodies are formed in the body against the antigen.

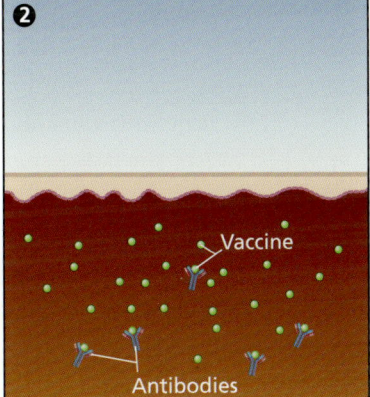

**Step 3:**

When the body is exposed to the organism against which the vaccine was directed, pre-made antibodies quickly help to fight the infection before it becomes established.

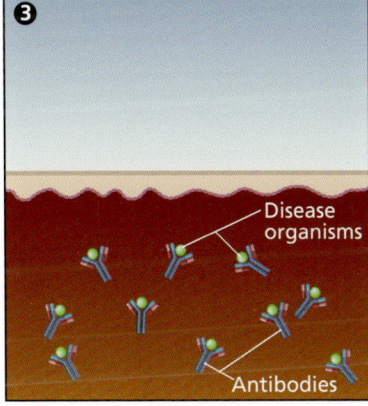

Exposing people to these diverse molecules will not only help their bodies develop several different types of antibodies, it will also make it more difficult for the *H. pylori* organism to develop changes that will allow it to escape the vaccine's activity. It is also important that the molecules used in the vaccination are not too similar to molecules that naturally occur in humans; otherwise, cross-reactive antibodies and autoimmune reactions may occur. Because different strains of *H. pylori* vary in the exact structure or types of proteins that they make, it has been difficult to find a single set of molecules that all strains make and that aren't too similar to normal human molecules.

Development of a vaccine is the most likely way to eradicate *H. pylori* from the human population. The expense of antibiotic therapy, on the other hand, is certain to restrict its use to wealthier countries that can afford it (typically the ones with lower rates of infection, who arguably need it less). A vaccine, which may cost only a few dollars per person, is likely to be a less expensive and more widely available alternative. Vaccines may also be less prone to resistance and negative side effects than the typical antibiotic-based treatments.

Where do we stand in the process of vaccine development? Currently experimental vaccines being developed in animal models are showing some promise, and there have been a few vaccine studies in humans. However, no vaccine is presently available, though it is probably just a matter of time before one is developed. Considering the number of people that *H. pylori* affects and the severity of the diseases that it can produce, an effective vaccine for *H. pylori* may dramatically improve the quality of human health worldwide.

**adaptive immune system (also called the acquired immune system)**—The branch of the immune system that responds to specific foreign molecules. It includes T and B cells, and antibodies (produced by B cells). The immune response produced by this system requires time to develop and occurs after exposure to the foreign molecule.

**adenocarcinoma**—A cancerous tumor originating in cells of a gland.

**adhesins**—Cell surface proteins expressed by *H. pylori* that bind to membrane-components (fats, sugars, and/or protiens) of the host's stomach cells. Adhesins promote attachment of the bacterial cell to the surface of the stomach.

**alimentary canal**—the tubular passage that extends from mouth to anus, functions in digestion and absorption of food and elimination of residual waste, and includes the mouth, throat, esophagus, stomach, small intestine, and large intestine.

**alpha-carbonic anhydrase (α-CA)**—An enzyme located in the space between the outer and inner membranes of *H. pylori* that converts carbon dioxide gas produced by the urease enzyme into bicarbonate, an acid-neutralizing compound.

**amino acids**—The building blocks from which proteins are constructed; they are also the end product of protein digestion.

**amylase**—Any of a group of enzymes that breaks down sugars.

**anecdotal evidence**—Evidence used to support a scientific argument. This kind of evidence is deficient because it is based on hearsay rather than a systematic collection of data.

**anemia**—A condition in which the blood is deficient in red blood cells or hemoglobin (the red, oxygen-carrying pigment in blood).

**antibodies (also called immunoglobulins)**—Any of a large number of proteins that are produced normally by specialized B cells after stimulation by a specific foreign molecule. Antibodies act specifically against the foreign molecule in an immune response, and may also be produced abnormally by some cancer cells.

**antigens**—Any substance that is foreign to the body and elicits an immune response, either alone or after combining with a larger molecule. Antigens are capable of binding with other products of the immune response (such as an antibody or a T cell).

**antrum**—The lower third of the stomach, near the small intestine.

**apoptosis (also called programmed cell death)**—A process of cellular self-destruction that is a normal physiological process aimed at eliminating damaged, unwanted cells. When apoptosis does not happen properly, uncontrolled cell growth and tumor formation may occur.

# Glossary

**aqueous**—Made from, with, or by water.

**arginase**—An enzyme that converts the amino acid L-arginine to urea.

**ascending colon**—The part of the large intestine that extends from the small intestine to the bend on the right side below the liver.

**auto-antibodies**—Proteins made by the immune system that target the cells or tissues of the individual producing them, damaging the tissue.

**autoimmune disease**—Diseases caused by antibodies or T cells that attack the organism's own molecules or cells.

**autoimmune neutropenia**—A condition in which antibodies, to mature neutrophils (a type of white blood cell), form, leading to cell destruction and a reduction in the blood's neutrophil count. This condition can cause an increased susceptibility to infection.

**autopsy (also called necropsy, postmortem, postmortem examination)**—An examination of the body after death, usually to expose the vital organs in order to determine the cause of death or the type of injury produced by a disease.

**BabA**—A protein on the outer membrane of the *H. pylori* organism that binds to the proteins on the outer membrane of many cells in the stomach. It is used by *H. pylori* to adhere to the stomach's lining.

**bile**—A greenish-yellow fluid that is made by the liver and stored in the gallbladder. It helps the intestines digest fat.

**body (of the stomach)**—The largest part of the stomach.

**bolus**—A mass of chewed food that is ready to be swallowed.

**brush border**—The lining of the small intestine, which is packed with small projecting structures (called microvilli) that give the tissue the microscopic appearance of a brush.

**CagA**—A toxic protein produced by *H. pylori* that injures the attachments between cells in the lining of the stomach, causing cells to detach from one another, thus damaging the tissue.

**capillaries**—Tiny blood vessels that supply tissue with oxygen and nutrients. In the intestine, they absorb nutrients and carry them to the circulatory system for distribution to the body's tissues.

**carbohydrates**—A group of organic molecules, including sugars and starches, that are composed of carbon, hydrogen, and oxygen atoms.

**carboxypeptidase**—A digestive enzyme made by the pancreas that breaks proteins into amino acids.

**carcinogen**—Any substance or physical agent that is capable of causing cancer.

**cardia**—The part of the stomach immediately adjacent to and surrounding the opening of the esophagus.

**chemotaxis (chemotactic behavior)**—A cell's response to the presence of a chemical. This response directs the cell's movement.

**chronic**—Of long duration; showing little change or slow progression.

**chyme**—The mixture of partially digested food and digestive secretions found in the stomach and small intestine during the digestion of a meal.

**chymotrypsin**—A digestive enzyme produced by the pancreas that functions within the small intestine to degrade proteins into amino acids.

**collagenase**—An enzyme that degrades collagen, a protein found in bones and connective tissue.

**common bile duct**—A tube that carries bile from the liver and gallbladder to the duodenum.

**complement**—A group of proteins in the blood that plays a vital role in the immune defenses. Complement proteins are inactive in the blood until activated by a foreign protein (e.g., a microbe) or another biochemical signal. Once activated, complement helps to eliminate the foreign molecule.

**cross-reaction**—A reaction between an antibody and another molecule produced by the host. This can occur when the host molecule is similar to a foreign molecule that the antibody was originally created to attack.

**cytokines**—Proteins secreted by white blood cells and certain other cells that provide signals to the immune system and regulate the immune function during immune responses.

**deglutition**—The act of swallowing.

**descending colon**—A portion of the large intestine (colon) that lies between the transverse colon and the rectum.

**duodenal ulcer**—A sore in the upper part of the small intestine (the duodenum).

**duodenum**—The part of the small intestine that connects the stomach and the jejunum (the upper part of the small intestine).

**ELISA (enzyme-linked immunosorbent assay)**—A test used as a general screening tool for the detection of specific substances related to the presence of an infectious organism.

**endoscope**—A device consisting of a tube and an optical system for observing the inside of a hollow organ such as the stomach.

**endotoxin**—A molecule (LPS) that is part of the cell wall of a gram-negative bacterium.

# Glossary

**enzyme**—A protein, produced by living organisms, that promotes chemical reactions between other substances without being consumed or destroyed by the reaction.

**epidemiologist**—A scientist who studies diseases in populations of people.

**epidemiology**—The study of the distribution of diseases in a population, the factors determining this distribution, and the application of this research to the control of health problems.

**epiglottis**—A lid-like structure made of cartilage that closes the opening to the lungs (glottis) while food or liquid is passing through the throat.

**eradicate**—To completely eliminate a disease-causing organism (such as *H. pylori*) from infected tissues or from a population.

**esophagus**—The muscular tube, about 10 to 12 inches (25 to 30 cm) in length, that carries swallowed food and liquids from the pharynx to the stomach.

**essential amino acids**—Amino acids (protein components) that an organism needs, and that must be supplied in its diet because they cannot be synthesized by the organism.

**extravasation**—The process of migration from a blood vessel into the tissues.

**feces**—Body waste, such as food residue, bacteria, epithelium, and mucus, discharged from the intestines. Also called excrement or stool.

**flagella**—Whip-like structures on the tail end of the *H. pylori* organism that enable it to move in the stomach.

**G cells**—Secretory cells found in the lining of the stomach that are responsible for the secretion of the hormone, gastrin.

**gall bladder**—A digestive organ that stores bile.

**gastric**—Relating to the stomach.

**gastric atrophy**—Also called *atrophic gastritis*. Prolonged or continual inflammation of the stomach lining that leads to changes in the tissue and results in a loss of acid and/or enzyme secretion.

**gastric lymphoma**—A type of cancer that can form in certain white blood cells in the stomach (B cells and T cells, primarily). Gastric lymphoma can spread to local lymph nodes, which can carry the disease throughout the body.

**gastric ulcer**—An open sore in the lining of the stomach.

**gastrin**—A group of hormones secreted by G cells in the stomach lining in response to mechanical stress or low acidity.

**gastritis**—Inflammation of the stomach lining that may result from infection with *H. pylori*, use of alcohol or tobacco, injury caused by certain medicines (such as aspirin), or autoimmune diseases.

**gastroesophageal sphincter**—A ring of smooth muscle fibers at the junction of the esophagus and stomach. Also called *cardiac sphincter*, or *lower esophageal sphincter*.

**gentian violet**—An antibacterial dye that is often painted on infected skin; also used in the Gram procedure to stain bacteria for observation on a microscope slide.

**gram-negative bacteria**—A common type of bacteria, normally found in the intestinal tract, that can be responsible for disease in humans. Bacteria are considered to be gram-negative because of their appearance under the microscope, where they either do not stain or are de-colorized by alcohol during the Gram staining procedure, and appear pink under a microscope.

**granules**—Small, grain-like masses inside of certain cells (such as neutrophils or macrophages) that can contain a variety of substances, including enzymes or other proteins.

**hemoglobin**—The oxygen-carrying pigment of the red blood cell.

**hydrogen peroxide**—A product of some immune cells that is used to kill invading bacteria.

**hypothesis**—A theory that can be scientifically tested and can therefore explain an observation or other phenomenon.

**ileocecal valve**—The valve through which contents of the small intestine pass into the large intestine.

**immune thrombocytopenia purpura (ITP)**— A disease in which the platelets (blood- clotting cells) of the blood are depleted by antibodies that bind to them and cause their destruction.

**inflamed**—The reaction of living tissues to injury, infection, or irritation; characterized by redness, heat, swelling, and pain.

**initiation**—The first stage of tumor induction by a chemical or physical agent that causes cancer. Initiation alters cells and makes them more likely to form a tumor.

**innate immune system**—The branch of the immune system that responds immediately to certain microbial threats. This response is not specific to the foreign molecule or microbe.

**interleukin-8 (IL-8)**—A protein that activates and attracts white blood cells during an immune response.

**intestinal metaplasia**—The abnormal transformation of tissue in the stomach lining that, under a microscope, gives it the appearance of intestinal tissue.

# Glossary

**jejunum**—The upper segment of the small intestine that lies between the duodenum and lower part of the small intestine (the ileum).

**Lewis b antigen**—A protein on the surface of many cells (blood cells, stomach cells, and others). Through its interaction with BabA, it may serve as a point of attachment of *H. pylori* to the stomach tissue.

**lingual lipase**—A digestive enzyme produced by the tongue that aids in the breakdown of fats.

**lipids**—Fats or fat-like substances.

**lipopolysaccharide (LPS)**—*See* Endotoxin.

**liver**—The largest solid organ in the body, it is situated in the upper right side of the abdomen, below the diaphragm. The liver is responsible for manufacturing a number of substances necessary for life, including complement, blood proteins, and bile.

**LPS**—*See* Endotoxin.

**lumen**—The cavity or channel within a tube or tubular organ.

**lymphocyte**—A white blood cell responsible for much of the body's immune protection. There are different subtypes, the most numerous of which are T and B cells.

**lymphoma**—A type of cancer derived from a type of white blood cell called a lymphocyte.

**macrophage**—A type of white blood cell found in the tissue that participates in the inflammatory process during an infection.

**malignant**—Cancerous.

**MALT lymphoma (mucosa-associated lymphoid tissue)**—A type of lymphoma that is found in the stomach.

**masticate**—To chew.

**metaplasia**—Conversion of tissue into a form that is not normal for that organ or tissue.

**metastasis**—Movement of cancer cells from one location to another, causing spread of the disease.

**microaerophilic culture**—A type of bacterial culture performed in the laboratory in special chambers that provide an atmosphere of low-oxygen content.

**microvilli**—Microscopic projections on the free surface of cell membranes in the intestinal lining. These projections greatly increase intestinal surface area and improve the efficiency of nutrient absorption during digestion.

**mitochondrion**—A structure inside of cells that is responsible for producing much of the cell's energy.

**mucin**—A protein found in mucus, which is present in saliva, bile, skin, glandular tissues, tendons, and cartilage.

**mucosa**—A moist tissue layer that lines the hollow organs and cavities of the body that open to the outside.

**mucous cells**—The cells of a type of membrane that covers organs and lines body cavities. These cells secrete mucus.

**multistage model of carcinogenesis**—The theory that cells become cancerous as a result of undergoing at least two types of injuries or changes (an initiation event followed by promotion).

**mutagen**—An agent that causes genetic mutations (changes).

**neutrophil**—A type of white blood cell that is responsible for much of the body's immune protection against infection.

**nitric oxide (NO)**—A soluble gas that is produced in the body by many cell types, including white blood cells.

**oncogene**—A gene that is usually very well regulated, but in unhealthy cells has the ability to induce a cell to become cancerous. Unregulated oncogenes may cause cells to grow and divide excessively.

**opsonization**—The attachment of certain proteins, such as antibodies and/or complement, to the surface of a foreign molecule or microbe, making that organism more susceptible to elimination by white blood cells.

**pancreas**—An organ in the abdominal cavity that produces digestive enzymes, insulin, and other hormones that regulate metabolism.

**pancreatic amylase**—An enzyme produced by the pancreas that aids in the digestion of carbohydrates.

**pancreatic lipase**—An enzyme produced by the pancreas that aids in the digestion of fats.

**parietal cells**—Cells of the gastric glands that secrete acid.

**pathogen**—An agent that causes disease.

**pathologist**—A physician who specializes in identifying diseases by studying cells and tissues under a microscope.

**pepsin**—An enzyme in the stomach that aids in the digestion of proteins.

**pepsinogen**—The inactive form of the digestive enzyme pepsin, which is produced by the stomach. Pepsinogen is converted to pepsin by exposure to stomach acid.

**peptidase**—A generic name for an enzyme that digests protein, also known as a *protease*.

**peptide bond**—The chemical linkage between two amino acids in a protein.

# Glossary

**peptides**—Small fragments of protein produced by the activity of enzymes that digest proteins.

**peptidoglycan**—A complex of polysaccharides and proteins found in the inner cell wall of bacteria.

**perforated ulcer**—A very deep ulcer that penetrates through the wall of the stomach, creating a hole through which stomach acid and stomach contents may leak into the abdominal cavity.

**peritonitis**—Inflammation of the abdominal cavity.

**periplasmic spaces**—The region between the plasma membrane and the cell wall of gram-negative bacteria.

**peristaltic waves**—The wormlike movements of the intestinal tract caused by contraction of muscle fibers. These movements propel the intestine's contents along the length of the organ.

**phagocytosis**—Ingestion of particles, such as microorganisms or fragments of cells. During phagocytosis material is taken into the cell in membrane-bound structures (phagosomes) that originate as pinched-off "bubbles" (vesicles) of the engulfing cell's outer membrane. Phagosomes fuse with other vesicles that contain enzymes, leading to degradation of the engulfed material.

**phagosome**—Membrane-bound "bubbles" (vesicles) that form inside of cells during the process of phagocytosis.

**pharynx**—The throat

**photosynthesis**—The process by which plants convert water and carbon dioxide into carbohydrate molecules.

**pili**—Hair-like projections on the surface of some bacteria that are involved in adhesion to surfaces and transfer of bacterial products between cells.

**progression**—The process by which tumors become increasingly cancerous.

**promotion**—Stimulation of tumor formation in a cell that has undergone a mutation, by an agent that promotes cell division.

**protease**—See *peptidase*.

**proton pumps**—Proteins on the surface of the parietal cells of the stomach that transport hydrogen ions (protons) across a membrane in exchange for potassium ions.

**pyloric sphincter**—A circular muscle layer between the bottom of the stomach and the opening of the small intestine that regulates the flow of stomach contents into the small intestine. Also called the *pylorus*.

**pylorus**—See *pyloric sphincter*.

**rectum**—The lower part of the large intestine, about 5 inches (12.7 cm) in length, that leads to the outside of the body via the anus.

**salivary amylase**—The digestive enzyme produced by the salivary glands that causes the breakdown of carbohydrates.

**salivary glands**—The numerous glands near the mouth that secrete saliva.

**sarcoma**—A cancer that arises from muscle or bone.

**statistics**—The collection, organization, and analysis of numerical data.

**stomach**—The portion of the digestive tract that is situated between the esophagus and the small intestine. It lies in the upper portion of the abdomen, to the left of the midline. The stomach produces acid and enzymes that help to break down food.

**tight junctions**—The junctions that seal adjacent cells together, and thereby prevent the passage of most molecules from one side of the cell layer to the other.

**trachea**—The windpipe. The tube that leads from the throat into the lungs.

**tumor suppressor**—A gene that normally regulates cell growth, and that is often mutated or otherwise inactivated when a cell becomes cancerous.

**trypsin**—An enzyme produced by the pancreas that digests protein into amino acids.

**urease**—An enzyme produced by *H. pylori* that converts urea into ammonia and $CO_2$ gas. This enzyme is crucial to the survival of *H. pylori* in the stomach, because the ammonia that it produces partially neutralizes the acidic environment that it would otherwise be unable to tolerate.

**VacA**—Vacuolating toxin A, a protein produced by *H. pylori*, which forms "bubbles," or vacuoles, in cells of the stomach lining. These bubbles cause cellular materials to be released, which provides *H. pylori* with nutrients, but damages tissue.

**vacuoles**—Bubble-like spaces within a cell that may contain various types of materials.

**villus (pl. villi)**—A small projection into the cavity of the small intestine that serves to increase the intestine's absorptive surface.

**viscous liquid**—A thick liquid.

# Additional Resources

ELECTRONIC RESOURCES

**BBC News**
http://news.bbc.co.uk
> Searching for the word "pylori" yields a number of nice news articles about this germ.

**The *Helicobacter* Foundation**
http://www.helico.com/
> Founded by Dr. Barry Marshall (one of the two discoverers of *H. pylori*), this Web site provides scientific information as well as an electronic discussion forum to discuss *H. pylori* and related diseases.

**Department of Bacteriology, University of Wisconsin-Madison**
http://www.bact.wisc.edu
> Dr. Karrie Holston's Web site is designed for use by her students, and provides a nice overview of the discovery of *H. pylori* and its diseases.

**KidsHealth**
http://kidshealth.org/
> Provides a nice introduction to ulcers and *H. pylori* for both parents and kids.

**Museum of Bacteria**
http://www.bacteriamuseum.org
> Provides many useful links about *H. pylori* on its *Helicobacter* Web page.

**Patient UK**
http://www.patient.co.uk
> This Web site has many helpful links for patients in the UK, as well as a few nice articles written for patients.

**U.S. Centers for Disease Control and Prevention (CDC)**
http://www.cdc.gov/
> Provides information about the symptoms, causes, and treatment of ulcers.

**U.S. National Digestive Diseases Information Clearinghouse (NIDDK)**
http://digestive.niddk.nih.gov/
> This Web site provides an excellent array of information about ulcers and *H. pylori*.

## PRINTED RESOURCES

Ben-Ari, Elia T. "New Take on Ulcer Bug Origins." *BioScience.* 50, no.7 (2000): 632.

    This brief article discusses the different strains of *H. pylori* and how the strains vary in different geographical regions.

Christensen, Damaris. "Is Your Stomach Bugging You?" *Science News.* 156, no.15 (1999): 234.

    This article discusses the discovery of *H. pylori* and the debate that still exists among health care workers about the value of eradicating this organism.

Fackelmann, Kathy. "Italians Discover Mouse Model for Ulcers." *Science News.* 147, no.11 (1995): 164.

    This article discusses the mouse model that was developed to study *H. pylori* and ulcer formation.

Hamilton, Gary. "Dead Man Walking." *New Scientist.* 171, no. 2303 (2001): 31.

    This article provides the history of Drs. Marshall and Warren, and their discovery of *H. pylori.*

Marshall, Barry, ed. *Helicobacter Pioneers: Firsthand Accounts from the Scientists Who Discovered Helicobacters, 1892-1982.* Victoria, Australia: Blackwell Publishing, 2002.

    Dr. Barry Marshall, one of the two physicians who discovered *H. pylori*, edited this book. While not an easy-read, the two articles by Drs. Marshall and Warren provide a detailed discussion of how they discovered the organism. Other chapters provide information about how the work of other scientists supported their ideas about the infectious origin of stomach ulcers.

Mestel, Rosie. "Sugary Clues to Stomach Ulcers." *New Scientist.* 141, no.1908 (1994): 15.

    This article discusses the role of the Lewis b antigens in *H. pylori* infection and disease formation.

Mlot, Christine. "Can Houseflies Spread the Ulcer Bacterium?" *Science News.* no. 40 (June 7, 1997): 350.

    This article discusses the scientific evidence for the idea that houseflies can spread *H. pylori.*

Richardson, Sarah. "Ulcers from Drinking?" *Discover.* 16, no. 10 (1995): 38.

    This article discusses the idea that drinking water can spread *H. pylori* in Colombia.

Sobel, Rachel K. "A Bane's Blessing." *U.S. News & World Report.* (January 14, 2002): 48.

# Additional Resources

This article talks about *H. pylori* and its relationship to gastric reflux disease. It proposes a controversial idea that *H. pylori* may prevent gastric reflux-related diseases.

Schubert, Charlotte. "Enzyme Defends Germ Against Stomach Acid." *Science News.* 59, no. 23 (2001): 358.
This brief article discusses the role of the *H. pylori* urease enzyme in the organism's ability to survive in the stomach.

Seppa, Nathan. "Did Colonization Spread Ulcers?" *Science News.* 157, no. 25 (2000): 395.
This article discusses the evidence for the idea that the colonization of the Americas caused the spread of *H. pylori* to the New World.

Travis, John. "A Flowery Toxin Reveals its Petals." *Science News.* 152, no.14 (1997): 218.
This article discusses the *H. pylori* VacA toxin and its role in disease.

——. "The Beast in the Belly" (BioBriefs) *BioScience.* 48, no. 7 (1998): 576.
This brief article discusses how attachment of *H. pylori* to the stomach lining affects disease formation.

Abbas, A.K., A.H. Lichtman, and J.S. Pober. *Cellular and Molecular Immunology,* 2nd Ed. Philadelphia: W.B. Saunders Company, 1994.

Aguemon, B. D., et al. "Prevalence and Risk-Factors for *Helicobacter pylori* Infection in Urban and Rural Beninese Populations." *Clinical Microbiology and Infection* 11, no. 8 (2005): 611–617.

Aguilar, G. R., G. Ayala, and G. Fierros-Zarate. "*Helicobacter pylori*: Recent Advances in the Study of Its Pathogenicity and Prevention." *Salud Pública de México* 43, no. 3 (2001): 237–247.

Amieva, M. R., et al. "*Helicobacter pylori* Enter and Survive within Multivesicular Vacuoles of Epithelial Cells." *Cellular Microbiology* 4, no. 10 (2002): 677–690.

Appelmelk, B. J., et al. "Potential Role of Molecular Mimicry between *Helicobacter pylori* Lipopolysaccharide and Host Lewis Blood Group Antigens in Autoimmunity." *Infection and Immunity* 64, no. 6 (1996): 2031–2040.

Arend, A., et al. "*Helicobacter pylori* Substantially Increases Oxidative Stress in Indomethacin-Exposed Rat Gastric Mucosa." *Medicina (Kaunas)* 41, no. 4 (2005): 343–347.

Ashbolt, N. J. "Microbial Contamination of Drinking Water and Disease Outcomes in Developing Regions." *Toxicology* 198, no. 1–3 (2004): 229–238.

Athmann, C., et al. "Local Ph Elevation Mediated by the Intrabacterial Urease of *Helicobacter pylori* Cocultured with Gastric Cells." *Journal of Clinical Investigation* 106, no. 3 (2000): 339–347.

Aviles-Jimenez, F., et al. "Evolution of the *Helicobacter pylori* Vacuolating Cytotoxin in a Human Stomach." *Journal of Bacteriology* 186, no. 15 (2004): 5182–5185.

Backstrom, A., et al. "Metastability of *Helicobacter pylori* Bab Adhesin Genes and Dynamics in Lewis B Antigen Binding." *Proceedings of the National Academy of Sciences, USA* 101, no. 48 (2004): 16923–16928.

Bardhan, P. K. "Epidemiological Features of *Helicobacter pylori* Infection in Developing Countries." *Clinical Infectious Diseases* 25, no. 5 (1997): 973–978.

Bergman, M. P., et al. "*Helicobacter pylori* Modulates the T Helper Cell 1/T Helper Cell 2 Balance through Phase-Variable Interaction between Lipopolysaccharide and Dc-Sign." *Journal of Experimental Medicine* 200, no. 8 (2004): 979–990.

———. "The Story So Far: *Helicobacter pylori* and Gastric Autoimmunity." *International Reviews of Immunology* 24, no. 1–2 (2005): 63–91.

# Bibliography

Betten, A., et al. "A Proinflammatory Peptide from *Helicobacter pylori* Activates Monocytes to Induce Lymphocyte Dysfunction and Apoptosis." *Journal of Clinical Investigation* 108, no. 8 (2001): 1221–1228.

Blanchard, T. G., M. L. Drakes, and S. J. Czinn. "*Helicobacter* Infection: Pathogenesis." *Current Opinion in Gastroenterology* 20, no. 1 (2004): 10–15.

Blaser, M. J. "Ecology of *Helicobacter pylori* in the Human Stomach." *Journal of Clinical Investigation* 100, no. 4 (1997): 759–762.

Blaser, M. J., and J. C. Atherton. "*Helicobacter pylori* Persistence: Biology and Disease." *Journal of Clinical Investigation* 113, no. 3 (2004): 321–333.

Bloom, W., and D. W. Fawcett,(ed.). *Textbook of Histology*, 11 ed. Philadelphia: W.B. Saunders Company, 1986.

Bobrzynski, A., et al. "*Helicobacter pylori* and Nonsteroidal Anti-Inflammatory Drugs in Perforations and Bleeding of Peptic Ulcers." *Medical Science Monitor* 11, no. 3 (2005): CR132–CR135.

Boyanova, L., et al. "Risk Factors for Primary *Helicobacter pylori* Resistance in Bulgarian Children." *Journal of Medical Microbiology* 53, Pt 9 (2004): 911–914.

Brock, T.D., D.W. Smith, and M.T. Madigan. *Biology of Microorganisms*, Fourth Edition. Englewood Cliffs, N.J.: Prentice-Hall, Inc., 1984.

Bytzer, P., and C. O'Morain. "Treatment of *Helicobacter pylori*." *Helicobacter* 10, Suppl 1 (2005): 40–46.

Campbell, D. I., et al. "Immunoglobulin G Subclass Responses to *Helicobacter pylori* Vary with Age in Populations with Different Levels of Risk of Gastric Carcinoma." *Clinical Diagnostic and Laboratory Immunology* 11, no. 3 (2004): 631–633.

Catalano, M., et al. "*Helicobacter pylori* Vaca Genotypes, CagA Status and Urea-B Polymorphism in Isolates Recovered from an Argentine Population." *Diagnostic Microbiology and Infectious Diseases* 41, no. 4 (2001): 205–210.

Chan, F. K., et al. "Preventing Recurrent Upper Gastrointestinal Bleeding in Patients with *Helicobacter pylori* Infection Who Are Taking Low-Dose Aspirin or Naproxen." *New England Journal of Medicine* 344, no. 13 (2001): 967–973.

Cheng, Y., et al. "*Helicobacter pylori*-Induced Macrophage Apoptosis Requires Activation of Ornithine Decarboxylase by C-Myc." *Journal of Biological Chemistry* 280, no. 23 (2005): 22492–22496.

Chiba, N., et al. "Treating *Helicobacter pylori* Infection in Primary Care Patients with Uninvestigated Dyspepsia: The Canadian Adult Dyspepsia

Empiric Treatment-*Helicobacter pylori* Positive (Cadet-Hp) Randomised Controlled Trial." *British Medical Journal* 324, no. 7344 (2002): 1012–1016.

———. "Economic Evaluation of *Helicobacter pylori* Eradication in the Cadet-Hp Randomized Controlled Trial of *H. Pylori*-Positive Primary Care Patients with Uninvestigated Dyspepsia." *Alimentary Pharmacology and Therapeutics* 19, no. 3 (2004): 349–358.

Cines, D. B., et al. "Congenital and Acquired Thrombocytopenia." *Hematology* (American Society of Hematology Education Program) (2004): 390–406.

Clyne, M., and B. Drumm. "The Urease Enzyme of *Helicobacter pylori* Does Not Function as an Adhesin." *Infection and Immunity* 64, no. 7 (1996): 2817–2820.

Covacci, A., and R. Rappuoli. "*Helicobacter pylori*: After the Genomes, Back to Biology." *Journal of Experimental Medicine* 197, no. 7 (2003): 807–811.

Croinin, T. O., M. Clyne, and B. Drumm. "Molecular Mimicry of Ferret Gastric Epithelial Blood Group Antigen a by *Helicobacter mustelae*." *Gastroenterology* 114, no. 4 (1998): 690–696.

Croinin, T. O., et al. "Antigastric Autoantibodies in Ferrets Naturally Infected with *Helicobacter mustelae*." *Infection and Immunity* 69, no. 4 (2001): 2708–2713.

Crowe, S. E. "*Helicobacter* Infection, Chronic Inflammation, and the Development of Malignancy." *Current Opinion in Gastroenterology* 21, no. 1 (2005): 32–38.

Cucinotta, F. A., and J. W. Wilson. "An Initiation-Promotion Model of Tumour Prevalence from High-Charge and Energy Radiations." *Physics in Medicine and Biology* 39, no. 11 (1994): 1811–1831.

D'Elios, M. M., et al. "Gastric Autoimmunity: The Role of *Helicobacter pylori* and Molecular Mimicry." *Trends in Molecular Medicine* 10, no. 7 (2004): 316–323.

de Jonge, R., et al. "Role of the *Helicobacter pylori* Outer-Membrane Proteins AlpA and AlpB in Colonization of the Guinea Pig Stomach." *Journal of Medical Microbiology* 53, Pt 5 (2004): 375–379.

De Luca, A., and G. Iaquinto. "*Helicobacter pylori* and Gastric Diseases: A Dangerous Association." *Cancer Letters* 213, no. 1 (2004): 1–10.

de Oliveira, A. M., et al. "Seroconversion for *Helicobacter pylori* in Adults from Brazil." *Transactions of the Royal Society of Tropical Medicine and Hygiene* 93, no. 3 (1999): 261–263.

Delaney, B., P. Moayyedi, and D. Forman. "*Helicobacter pylori* Infection." *Clinical Evidence* 12 (2004): 641–658.

# Bibliography

Delaney, B., P. Moayyedi, and D. Forman. "*Helicobacter pylori* Infection." *Clinical Evidence* 13 (2005): 518–534.

Dubreuil, J.D., et al. "Effect of Heparin Binding on *Helicobacter pylori* Resistance to Serum." *Journal of Medical Microbiology* 53, Pt 1 (2004): 9–12.

Elitsur, Y., and J. Yahav. "*Helicobacter pylori* Infection in Pediatrics." *Helicobacter* 10, Suppl 1 (2005): 47–53.

Faber, J., et al. "Treatment Regimens for *Helicobacter pylori* Infection in Children: Is in Vitro Susceptibility Testing Helpful?" *Journal of Pediatric Gastroenterology and Nutrition* 40, no. 5 (2005): 571–574.

Fennerty, M.B. "*Helicobacter pylori*: Why It Still Matters in 2005." *Cleveland Clinic Journal of Medicine* 72, Suppl 2 (2005): S1–7; discussion S14–S21.

Forman, D., and D. Y. Graham. "Review Article: Impact of *Helicobacter pylori* on Society-Role for a Strategy of 'Search and Eradicate.'" *Alimentary Pharmacology and Therapeutics* 19, Suppl 1 (2004): 17–21.

Fox, J. G., and T. C. Wang. "*Helicobacter pylori*—Not a Good Bug after All!" *New England Journal of Medicine* 345, no. 11 (2001): 829–832.

Genta, R.M. "The Gastritis Connection: Prevention and Early Detection of Gastric Neoplasms." *Journal of Clinical Gastroenterology* 36, 5 Suppl (2003): S44–S49; discussion S61–S62.

Gold, B. D., et al. "*Helicobacter pylori* Infection in Children: Recommendations for Diagnosis and Treatment." *Journal of Pediatric Gastroenterology and Nutrition* 31, no. 5 (2000): 490–497.

Gologan, A., D. Y. Graham, and A. R. Sepulveda. "Molecular Markers in *Helicobacter pylori*-Associated Gastric Carcinogenesis." *Clinical Laboratory Medicine* 25, no. 1 (2005): 197–222.

Goodman, K. J., and M. Cockburn. "The Role of Epidemiology in Understanding the Health Effects of *Helicobacter pylori*." *Epidemiology* 12, no. 2 (2001): 266–271.

Graham, D. Y. "NSAIDs, *Helicobacter pylori*, and Pandora's Box." *New England Journal of Medicine* 347, no. 26 (2002): 2162–2164.

Guiney, D. G., P. Hasegawa, and S. P. Cole. "*Helicobacter pylori* Preferentially Induces Interleukin 12 (Il–12) Rather Than Il–6 or Il–10 in Human Dendritic Cells." *Infection and Immunity* 71, no. 7 (2003): 4163–4166.

Gupta, V., A. J. Eden, and M. J. Mills. "*Helicobacter pylori* and Autoimmune Neutropenia." *Clinical and Laboratory Haematology* 24, no. 3 (2002): 183–185.

Guyton, A.C. *Textbook of Medical Physiology*. Philadelphia: W.B. Saunders Company, 1986.

Ha, N. C., et al. "Supramolecular Assembly and Acid Resistance of *Helicobacter pylori* Urease." *Nature Structural and Molecular Biology* 8, no. 6 (2001): 505–509.

Hennekens, C.H., and J.E. Buring *Epidemiology in Medicine*, 1st Ed. Boston: Little Brown and Company, 1987.

Hennig, E. E., et al. "Heterogeneity among *Helicobacter pylori* Strains in Expression of the Outer Membrane Protein Baba." *Infection and Immunity* 72, no.6 (2004): 3429–3435.

Henriksen, T. H. "Peptic Ulcer Disease Is Strongly Associated with *Helicobacter pylori* in East, West, Central and South Africa." *Scandinavian Journal of Gastroenterology* 36, no. 6 (2001): 561–564.

Imrie, C., et al. "Is *Helicobacter pylori* Infection in Childhood a Risk Factor for Gastric Cancer?" *Pediatrics* 107, no. 2 (2001): 373–380.

Ishikawa, N., et al. "*Helicobacter pylori* Infection in Rheumatoid Arthritis: Effect of Drugs on Prevalence and Correlation with Gastroduodenal Lesions." *Rheumatology* (Oxford) 41, no. 1 (2002): 72–77.

Ismail, S., M. B. Hampton, and J. I. Keenan. "*Helicobacter pylori* Outer Membrane Vesicles Modulate Proliferation and Interleukin-8 Production by Gastric Epithelial Cells." *Infection and Immunity* 71, no. 10 (2003): 5670–5675.

Isomoto, H., et al. "Enhanced Expression of Interleukin-8 and Activation of Nuclear Factor Kappa-B in Endoscopy-Negative Gastroesophageal Reflux Disease." *American Journal of Gastroenterology* 99, no. 4 (2004): 589–597.

Jacobs, S., and V. Falk. "Pearls and Pitfalls: Lessons Learned in Endoscopic Robotic Surgery—the Da Vinci Experience." *Heart Surgery Forum* 4, no. 4 (2001): 307–310.

Jang, J., et al. "Malgun (Clear) Cell Change in *Helicobacter pylori* Gastritis Reflects Epithelial Genomic Damage and Repair." *American Journal of Pathology* 162, no. 4 (2003): 1203–1211.

Kalach, N., et al. "*Helicobacter pylori* Infection Is Not Associated with Specific Symptoms in Nonulcer-Dyspeptic Children." *Pediatrics* 115, no. 1 (2005): 17–21.

Kamiji, M. M., and R. B. de Oliveira. "Non-Antibiotic Therapies for *Helicobacter pylori* Infection." *European Journal of Gastroenterology and Hepatology* 17, no. 9 (2005): 973–981.

# Bibliography

Kapadia, C. R. "Gastric Atrophy, Metaplasia, and Dysplasia: A Clinical Perspective." *Journal of Clinical Gastroenterology* 36, no. 5 Suppl (2003): S29–36; discussion S61–S62.

Kersulyte, D., et al. "Differences in Genotypes of *Helicobacter pylori* from Different Human Populations." *Journal of Bacteriology* 182, no. 11 (2000): 3210–3218.

Kikuchi, S., and M. P. Dore "Epidemiology of *Helicobacter pylori* Infection." *Helicobacter* 10, Suppl 1 (2005): 1–4.

Koch, A., et al. "Seroprevalence and Risk Factors for *Helicobacter pylori* Infection in Greenlanders." *Helicobacter* 10, no. 5 (2005): 433–442.

Kountouras, J., C. Zavos, and D. Chatzopoulos. "A Concept on the Role of *Helicobacter pylori* Infection in Autoimmune Pancreatitis." *Journal of Cellular and Molecular Medicine* 9, no. 1 (2005): 196–207.

Kranzer, K., et al. "Induction of Maturation and Cytokine Release of Human Dendritic Cells by *Helicobacter pylori.*" *Infection and Immunity* 72, no. 8 (2004): 4416–4423.

Krogfelt, K. A., P. Lehours, and F. Megraud. "Diagnosis of *Helicobacter pylori* Infection." *Helicobacter* 10, Suppl 1 (2005): 5–13.

Kuipers, E. J., and P. Michetti. "Bacteria and Mucosal Inflammation of the Gut: Lessons from *Helicobacter pylori.*" *Helicobacter* 10, Suppl 1 (2005): 66–70.

Kupcinskas, L., and P. Malfertheiner. "*Helicobacter pylori* and Non-Malignant Diseases." *Helicobacter* 10, Suppl 1 (2005): 26–33.

Ladeira, M. S., et al. "DNA Damage in Patients Infected by *Helicobacter pylori.*" *Cancer Epidemiology, Biomarkers and Prevention* 13, no. 4 (2004): 631–637.

Lo, C. C., et al. "Implications of Anti-Parietal Cell Antibodies and Anti-*Helicobacter pylori* Antibodies in Histological Gastritis and Patient Outcome." *World Journal of Gastroenterology* 11, no. 30 (2005): 4715–4720.

Lodish, H., D. Baltimore, A. Berk, S. L. Zipursky, P. Matsudaira, P., J. Darnell *Molecular Cell Biology*, 3rd ed. New York: W.H. Freeman, 1995.

Logan, R. P., and M. M. Walker. "ABC of the Upper Gastrointestinal Tract: Epidemiology and Diagnosis of *Helicobacter pylori* Infection." *British Medical Journal* 323, no. 7318 (2001): 920–922.

Lu, A. P., et al. "Correlation between Cd4, Cd8 Cell Infiltration in Gastric Mucosa, *Helicobacter pylori* Infection and Symptoms in Patients with Chronic Gastritis." *World Journal of Gastroenterology* 11, no. 16 (2005): 2486–2490.

Makristathis, A., et al. "Diagnosis of *Helicobacter pylori* Infection." *Helicobacter* 9, Suppl 1 (2004): 7–14.

Malaty, H. M., et al. "Age at Acquisition of *Helicobacter pylori* Infection: A Follow-up Study from Infancy to Adulthood." *Lancet* 359, no. 9310 (2002): 931–935.

Marcus, E. A., et al. "The Periplasmic Alpha-Carbonic Anhydrase Activity of *Helicobacter pylori* Is Essential for Acid Acclimation." *Journal of Bacteriology* 187, no. 2 (2005): 729–738.

Marshall, B., ed. Helicobacter *Pioneers: Firsthand Accounts from the Scientists Who Discovered Helicobacters, 1892–1982.* Victoria, Australia: Blackwell Publishing, 2002.

Maury, E., et al. "An Observational Study of Upper Gastrointestinal Bleeding in Intensive Care Units: Is *Helicobacter pylori* the Culprit?" *Critical Care Medicine* 33, no. 7 (2005): 1513–1518.

Megraud, F., et al. "Seroepidemiology of *Campylobacter pylori* Infection in Various Populations." *Journal of Clinical Microbiology* 27, no. 8 (1989): 1870–1873.

Megraud, F. "*H. pylori* Antibiotic Resistance: Prevalence, Importance, and Advances in Testing." *Gut* 53.9 (2004): 1374–1384.

———. "Basis for the Management of Drug-Resistant *Helicobacter pylori* Infection." *Drugs* 64, no. 17 (2004): 1893–1904.

Menaker, R. J., P. J. Ceponis, and N. L. Jones. "*Helicobacter pylori* Induces Apoptosis of Macrophages in Association with Alterations in the Mitochondrial Pathway." *Infection and Immunity* 72, no. 5 (2004): 2889–2898.

Meyer, F., et al. "Cutting Edge: Cyclooxygenase-2 Activation Suppresses Th1 Polarization in Response to *Helicobacter pylori.*" *Journal of Immunology* 171, no. 8 (2003): 3913–3917.

Michetti, P. "Vaccine against *Helicobacter pylori*: Fact or Fiction?" *Gut* 41, no. 6 (1997): 728–730.

———. "Development of a Vaccine against *Helicobacter pylori* Infection." *Italian Journal of Gastroenterology and Hepatology* 30, Suppl 3 (1998): S339–S341.

Mobley, H., Mendz, G. Hazell, S., ed. Helicobacter pylori: *Physiology and Genetics.* Washington, D.C.: ASM Press, 2001.

Modlin, I.M., and G. Sachs. *The Logic of Omeprazole: Treatment by Design.* Philadelphia: CoMed Communications, Inc., 2000.

# Bibliography

Monack, D. M., A. Mueller, and S. Falkow. "Persistent Bacterial Infections: The Interface of the Pathogen and the Host Immune System." *Nature Reviews. Microbiology* 2, no. 9 (2004): 747–765.

Monteiro, M. A., et al. "Simultaneous Expression of Type 1 and Type 2 Lewis Blood Group Antigens by *Helicobacter pylori* Lipopolysaccharides. Molecular Mimicry between *H. pylori* Lipopolysaccharides and Human Gastric Epithelial Cell Surface Glycoforms." *Journal of Biological Chemistry* 273, no.19 (1998): 11533–11543.

Moran, A. P., et al. "Phenotypic Variation in Molecular Mimicry between *Helicobacter pylori* Lipopolysaccharides and Human Gastric Epithelial Cell Surface Glycoforms. Acid–Induced Phase Variation in Lewis(X) and Lewis(Y) Expression by *H. Pylori* Lipopolysaccharides." *Journal of Biological Chemistry* 277, no. 8 (2002): 5785–5795.

Nguyen, T. N., A. N. Barkun, and C. A. Fallone. "Host Determinants of *Helicobacter pylori* Infection and Its Clinical Outcome." *Helicobacter* 4, no. 3 (1999): 185–197.

Ning, P. F., H. J. Liu, and Y. Yuan. "Dynamic Expression of Pepsinogen C in Gastric Cancer, Precancerous Lesions and *Helicobacter pylori* Associated Gastric Diseases." *World Journal of Gastroenterology* 11, no.17 (2005): 2545–2548.

Northfield, T.C., Mendall, M., Goggin, P.M., ed. Helicobacter pylori *Infection*. Dordrecht: Kluwer Academic Publishers, 1993.

O'Connor, H., and S. Sebastian. "The Burden of *Helicobacter pylori* Infection in Europe." *Alimentary Pharmacology and Therapeutics* 18, Suppl 3 (2003): 38–44.

Odze, R. D. "Unraveling the Mystery of the Gastroesophageal Junction: A Pathologist's Perspective." *American Journal of Gastroenterology* 100, no. 8 (2005): 1853–1867.

Oh, J. D., S. M. Karam, and J. I. Gordon. "Intracellular *Helicobacter pylori* in Gastric Epithelial Progenitors." *Proceedings of the National Academy of Science, USA* 102, no. 14 (2005): 5186–5191.

Ohkusa, T., T. Nomura, and N. Sato. "The Role of Bacterial Infection in the Pathogenesis of Inflammatory Bowel Disease." *Internal Medicine* 43, no. 7 (2004): 534–539.

Oliveira, A. G., et al. "BabA2- and CagA-Positive *Helicobacter pylori* Strains Are Associated with Duodenal Ulcer and Gastric Carcinoma in Brazil." *Journal of Clinical Microbiology* 41, no. 8 (2003): 3964–3966.

Osato, M. S., et al. "Pattern of Primary Resistance of *Helicobacter pylori* to Metronidazole or Clarithromycin in the United States." *Archives of Internal Medicine* 161, no. 9 (2001): 1217–1220.

Parsonnet, J. "Bacterial Infection as a Cause of Cancer." *Environmental Health Perspectives* 103, Suppl 8 (1995): 263–268.

Parsonnet, J., and P. G. Isaacson. "Bacterial Infection and Malt Lymphoma." *New England Journal of Medicine* 350, no. 3 (2004): 213–215.

Parsonnet, J., and D. Forman. "*Helicobacter pylori* Infection and Gastric Cancer—for Want of More Outcomes." *Journal of the American Medical Association* 291, no. 2 (2004): 244–245.

Permin, H., and L. P. Andersen. "Inflammation, Immunity, and Vaccines for *Helicobacter* Infection." *Helicobacter* 10, Suppl 1 (2005): 21–25.

Playfair, J.H.L., and P.M. Lydyard. *Medical Immunology for Students.* Edinburgh: Churchill Livingstone, 1995.

Ramarao, N., and T. F. Meyer. "*Helicobacter pylori* Resists Phagocytosis by Macrophages: Quantitative Assessment by Confocal Microscopy and Fluorescence-Activated Cell Sorting." *Infection and Immunity* 69, no. 4 (2001): 2604–2611.

Rautelin, H., P. Lehours, and F. Megraud. "Diagnosis of *Helicobacter pylori* Infection." *Helicobacter* 8, Suppl 1 (2003): 13–20.

Rautelin, H., and T. U. Kosunen. "*Helicobacter pylori* Infection in Finland." *Annals of Internal Medicine* 36, no. 2 (2004): 82–88.

Rektorschek, M., et al. "Acid Resistance of *Helicobacter pylori* Depends on the Urei Membrane Protein and an Inner Membrane Proton Barrier." *Molecular Microbiology* 36, no. 1 (2000): 141–152.

Robbins, S.L., R.S. Cotran, and V. Kumar. *Pathologic Basis of Disease.* Philadelphia: W.B. Saunders Company, 1995.

Rodrigues, M. N., et al. "Prevalence of *Helicobacter pylori* Infection in Fortaleza, Northeastern Brazil." *Revista de Saúde Pública* 39.5 (2005): 847–849.

Rokita, E., et al. "*Helicobacter pylori* Urease Significantly Reduces Opsonization by Human Complement." *Journal of Infectious Disease* 178, no. 5 (1998): 1521–1525.

Rothenbacher, D., G. Bode, and H. Brenner. "Dynamics of *Helicobacter pylori* Infection in Early Childhood in a High-Risk Group Living in Germany: Loss of Infection Higher Than Acquisition." *Alimentary Pharmacology and Therapeutics* 16, no. 9 (2002): 1663–1668.

# Bibliography

Ruddon, R.W. *Cancer Biology*, 3rd ed. New York: Oxford University Press, 1995.

Sachs, G., et al. "The Gastric Biology of *Helicobacter pylori*." *Annual Review of Physiology* 65 (2003): 349–369.

Scott, D., et al. "The Life and Death of *Helicobacter pylori*." *Gut* 43, Suppl 1 (1998): S56–S60.

Segni, M., et al. "Early Manifestations of Gastric Autoimmunity in Patients with Juvenile Autoimmune Thyroid Diseases." *Journal of Clinical Endocrinology and Metabolism* 89, no. 10 (2004): 4944–4948.

Shang, J., and A. S. Pena. "Multidisciplinary Approach to Understand the Pathogenesis of Gastric Cancer." *World Journal of Gastroenterology* 11, no. 27 (2005): 4131–4139.

Sheu, B. S., et al. "Host Gastric Lewis Expression Determines the Bacterial Density of *Helicobacter pylori* in BabA2 Genopositive Infection." *Gut* 52.7 (2003): 927–932.

Sinha, S. K., et al. "Age at Acquisition of *Helicobacter pylori* in a Pediatric Canadian First Nations Population." *Helicobacter* 7, no. 2 (2002): 76–85.

———. "The Incidence of *Helicobacter pylori* Acquisition in Children of a Canadian First Nations Community and the Potential for Parent-to-Child Transmission." *Helicobacter* 9, no. 1 (2004): 59–68.

Smellie, W. S., et al. "Best Practice in Primary Care Pathology: Review 1." *Journal of Clinical Pathology* 58, no.10 (2005): 1016–1024.

Sotoudehmanesh, R., et al. "Peptic Ulcer Bleeding: Is *Helicobacter pylori* a Risk Factor in an Endemic Area?" *Indian Journal of Gastroenterology* 24, no. 2 (2005): 59–61.

Suerbaum, S., and P. Michetti. "*Helicobacter pylori* Infection." *New England Journal of Medicine* 347, no. 15 (2002): 1175–1186.

Sugiyama, T., and M. Asaka. "*Helicobacter pylori* Infection and Gastric Cancer." *Medical Electron Microscopy* 37, no. 3 (2004): 149–157.

Sung, J. J., et al. "Cyclooxygenase-2 Expression in *Helicobacter pylori*-Associated Premalignant and Malignant Gastric Lesions." *American Journal of Pathology* 157, no. 3 (2000): 729–735.

Suzuki, H., et al. "Ammonia-Induced Apoptosis Is Accelerated at Higher pH in Gastric Surface Mucous Cells." *American Journal of Physiology: Gastrointestinal and Liver Physiology* 283, no. 4 (2002): G986–G995.

Talley, N. J., and N. Vakil. "Guidelines for the Management of Dyspepsia." *American Journal of Gastroenterology* 100, no. 10 (2005): 2324–2337.

Tang, Y. L., et al. "Detection and Location of *Helicobacter pylori* in Human Gastric Carcinomas." *World Journal of Gastroenterology* 11, no. 9 (2005): 1387–1391.

Terres, A. M., et al. "*Helicobacter pylori* Disrupts Epithelial Barrier Function in a Process Inhibited by Protein Kinase C Activators." *Infection and Immunity* 66, no. 6 (1998): 2943–2950.

Tham, K. T., et al. "*Helicobacter pylori* Genotypes, Host Factors, and Gastric Mucosal Histopathology in Peptic Ulcer Disease." *Human Pathology* 32, no. 3 (2001): 264–273.

Thomas, C.G.A. *Medical Microbiology,* Bailliere's Concise Medical Textbooks, 5th ed. London: Bailliere Tindall, 1983.

Tomasi, P. A., et al. "Is There Anything to the Reported Association between *Helicobacter pylori* Infection and Autoimmune Thyroiditis?" *Digestive Diseases and Sciences* 50, no. 2 (2005): 385–388.

Tortora, G.J., and N.P. Anagnostakos. *Principles of Anatomy and Physiology.* New York: Harper and Row Publishers, 1981.

Tummala, S., S. Keates, and C. P. Kelly. "Update on the Immunologic Basis of *Helicobacter pylori* Gastritis." *Current Opinions in Gastroenterology* 20, no. 6 (2004): 592–597.

Uibo, R. "Contribution of Epidemiological Studies to Gastritis Immunology." *International Reviews of Immunology* 24, no.1–2 (2005): 31–54.

Vakil, N., and A. M. Fendrick. "How to Test for *Helicobacter pylori* in 2005." *Cleveland Clinic Journal of Medicine* 72, Suppl 2 (2005): S8–13; discussion S14–S21.

Venes, D., ed. *Taber's Cyclopedic Medical Dictionary,* 20th ed. Philadelphia: F.A. Davis, 2005.

Versalovic, J. "*Helicobacter pylori.* Pathology and Diagnostic Strategies." *American Journal of Clinical Pathology* 119, no. 3 (2003): 403–412.

Vilaichone, R. K., et al. "Molecular Epidemiology and Outcome of *Helicobacter pylori* Infection in Thailand: A Cultural Cross Roads." *Helicobacter* 9, no. 5 (2004): 453–459.

Wang, L. L., et al. "Detection of T Lymphocyte Subsets of Children with *Helicobacter pylori* Infection." *World Journal of Gastroenterology* 11, no. 18 (2005): 2827–2829.

Webb, P. M., et al. "Gastric Cancer, Gastritis and Plasma Vitamin C: Results from an International Correlation and Cross-Sectional Study. The Eurogast Study Group." *International Journal of Cancer* 73, no. 5 (1997): 684–689.

# Bibliography

Weeks, D. L., et al. "Mechanism of Proton Gating of a Urea Channel." *Journal of Biological Chemistry* 279, no. 11 (2004): 9944–9950.

Wen, Y., et al. "Acid-Adaptive Genes of *Helicobacter pylori*." *Infection and Immunity* 71, no. 10 (2003): 5921–5939.

Wong, B. C., C. K. Ching, and S. K. Lam. "*Helicobacter pylori* Infection and Gastric Cancer." *Hong Kong Medical Journal* 5, no. 2 (1999): 175–179.

Xia, H. H., et al. "Macrophage Migration Inhibitory Factor Stimulated by *Helicobacter pylori* Increases Proliferation of Gastric Epithelial Cells." *World Journal of Gastroenterology* 11.13 (2005): 1946–50.

# Index

# Index

# Index

# About the Author

Shawna L. Fleming earned her bachelor's degree in Biology from the University of California, Riverside and her Ph.D. degree in Pathobiology from Brown University. She is currently employed in the Drug Safety Assessment Department at Synta Pharmaceuticals, in Lexington, Massachusetts.

# About the Editor

The late I. Edward Alcamo was a Distinguished Teaching Professor of Microbiology at the State University of New York at Farmingdale. Alcamo studied biology at Iona College in New York and earned his M.S. and Ph.D. degrees in microbiology at St. John's University, also in New York. He had taught at Farmingdale for more than 30 years. In 2000, Alcamo won the Carski Award for Distinguished Teaching in Microbiology, the highest honor for microbiology teachers in the United States. He was a member of the American Society for Microbiology, the National Association of Biology teachers, and the American Medical Writers Association. Alcamo authored numerous books on the subjects of microbiology, AIDS, and DNA technology as well as the award-winning textbook *Fundamentals of Microbiology*, now in its sixth edition.